When AIDS meets poverty

When AIDS meets poverty

Implications for social capital in a village in Tanzania

AWLAE SERIES No. 5

Carolyne I. Nombo

Wageningen Academic
Publishers

ISBN 978-90-8686-063-0

First published, 2007

Wageningen Academic Publishers
The Netherlands, 2007

Acknowledgement

This research for this publication was supported and funded by various organisations and people. The Netherlands Ministry of Foreign Affairs (DGIS), Winrock International - AWLAE team in Nairobi, Wageningen and the United States, your technical, logistical and financial support for this PhD study is highly acknowledged. I thank you all for having a confidence in me. I honour the late Prof. Julia Gitobu who sadly could not live to witness the reward for her dedication to the cause of African women leadership and the results of all the work she invested in the AWLAE Project. I would also like to express my deep sense of gratitude to the Mkamba community for allowing me to live and learn from them. Thanks for your assistance and information. Special thanks go to all those in Mkamba village who took time to meeting me, be interviewed, and share resources and ideas on my study.

A very special thanks to my academic supervisor (promotor) Prof. Anke Niehof for her professional advice, encouragement and timely advice wherever required. Your stimulating scientific discussions helped me all the time of research, without them it would not have been possible for me to accomplish the task. You made yourself available even through heavy teaching and travel workload. Through you I learnt to believe in my work and myself. Our relation transcended the academic sphere and included helping my family settle in the UK. I am deeply indebted to Dr. Bridget O'Laughlin, my co-promotor, for her detailed review, constructive criticism and extensive comments during the preparation of the publication to enhance its quality and improve my writing. I am greatly indebted to Prof. Amon Mattee my mentor who not only strongly recommended me for PhD studies but also offered enormous technical and moral support during the entire period. I appreciate your working style which promotes self-confidence and autonomy. I am most grateful to Dr. Lisa Price for her scientific guidance on gender issues during the first months of my studies in Wageningen. This exposure made a lot of difference to my thinking and writing. Thank you, Dr. Hester Moerbeek, for your guidance on matters of data analysis.

I enjoyed the company and the logistical support given by other members of Sociology of Consumers and Household Group. I thank you all for the critical solidarity. Hedy and Riet are especially thanked for their care and attention. You both made a huge contribution towards my settling and living in Wageningen by arranging all the formalities and always providing help when needed. Dinie, thank you for your excellent work on formatting the manuscript and turning it into a readable publication. Thanks Exuad Minja for your assistance with data entry, Mrs Mhina for transcription, and Alfred Chonya and Betty Mhando for translation of field materials. Thank you, Roy Jordaan, for the critical editing of the manuscript. Special thanks go to Robert,

Stephen Mguluka, Philipina Nyaki and Ngella, Suzanne Mbaki and Rausa Kaganda, my research assistants and good friends during my fieldwork in Mkamba.

It was rewarding to be in the company of cherished colleagues from different social groups in Wageningen like Wabongo, UTAKE, the Student Chaplaincy, the Seventh Day Adventist Group, ICF-International, and the Amazing Grace Parish. You gave me an unique experience in Wageningen. I was extremely fortunate to have the support of other special friends to whom I am truly grateful. My fellow ladies in AWLAE program supported me in different ways. I want to thank them for all their help, support, interest and the valuable time we had together. A journey is easier when you travel together; you all made my journey easier. Especially I am obliged to Faith Nguthi who was of great help in difficulties. Sharing an office with her was a blessing. Doris, I will always cherish our friendship. Thanks for your selfless support. I owe gratitude to Gaynor who provided me with support, encouragement and sound advice. I am grateful to Joyce Challe for being a constant source of inspiration and great help. I owe a lot to Marian Koster and Kidist Gebreselassi who provided valuable feedback to one of my papers. Thanks to Suzana Akrofi and Monica Karuhanga for their homely warmth in the Schaepmanstraat house, and to my host family friends Henk, Hester and the family, for their company in Wageningen.

My deep sense of gratitude goes to my parents Victoria and Ignatius who raised me, loved me and supported me and also taught me the value of hard work. You are the foundation of my vision. My brothers and sisters, Charles, Rosemary, Anneth and Peter provided me with strength to go on while you were ready to look after our sick mother. You are a real part of my achievement. Without your encouragement and support it would have not been possible to finish this work. I lack words of appreciation for Mussa Mtoni, my brother-in-law's family. You were very supportive; how can one leave one's own family and look after someone else's family? Mama Khalid you are more than a sister; you have taught me the value of sisterhood. To the other family members: thank you for your loving support and encouragement.

I owe my loving thanks to my husband Paul. Two PhDs endeavours in one household was not easy, but your patience, understanding and love made my dream come true. Thank you Paul, despite the academic pressure you dedicated time to discuss and read my drafts. Most importantly my deepest appreciation goes to you for assuming a motherly role to our boys when I was away. To our sons Tito and Timoth, your daily little prayer for dad and mum's studies made a lot of difference. You have endured my absence and less attention because of my study. Thank you for your understanding when I was not there for you.

It is not easy to mention everyone here but I appreciate and thank all who directly or indirectly helped the completion of this work. I cannot end without thanking God whose grace and blessing enabled me to realize this work. I return all the glory and honour to him.

Table of contents

Acknowledgement **7**

List of acronyms **15**

Glossary **17**

Chapter 1 Introduction **19**
1.1 Motivation for the study 19
1.2 HIV/AIDS situation in the country 19
1.3 Government responses to HIV/AIDS epidemic 22
1.4 Research problem and questions 24
1.5 Structure of the publication 26

Chapter 2 Household, livelihood, social capital and HIV/AIDS impacts: a conceptual and analytical framework **29**
2.1 Household 31
2.1.1 Intra-household differentiation 32
2.1.2 Kinship and inter-household relations 35
2.2 The livelihood framework 38
2.2.1 Household production of care 40
2.2.2 Household food security and its determinants 42
2.2.3 Livelihood vulnerability 44
2.2.4. Coping strategies 50
2.2.5 Collective arrangements and safety nets 53
2.3 Social capital 56
2.4 Conceptual framework of the study 65

Chapter 3 Research design and methodology **67**
3.1 Study site 67
3.2 Research design 68
3.2.1 Longitudinal approach 68
3.2.2 Combining qualitative and quantitative methods 68
3.3 Research units 69
3.4 Definition of HIV/AIDS cases 69
3.5 Data collection methods 70
3.5.1 Methods of primary data collection 70
3.5.2 Recruitment of research assistants 78
3.5.3 Secondary data collection 79
3.6 Data analysis 79

3.7 Validity and reliability 80
3.8 Discrepancies and methodological problems 81
3.9 Ethical considerations 82
3.10 Time schedule of the research 83

Chapter 4 Study area and context **85**
4.1 Basic health and HIV/AIDS services in Tanzania 85
4.2 The HIV/AIDS situation in Morogoro region 89
4.3 Kilombero District 91
4.4 Settlement patterns and village governance in Tanzania 93
4.5 Mkamba village 95
4.5.1 Socio-economic and demographic characteristics 95
4.5.2 Basic services 98
4.5.3 Households in Mkamba village 100
4.5.4 Social and community life in the village 101
4.5.5 A livelihood profile 106
4.5.6 History and significance of the sugar plantation in the area 109
4.5.7 Wealth profile of households in the village 114
4.6 Concluding notes 114

Chapter 5 Economic and social impacts of HIV/AIDS at the household level **117**
5.1 Characteristics of the respondents 117
5.2 The impact of HIV/AIDS on household assets and livelihood activities 121
5.2.1 Effects on human capital 121
5.2.2 Impact on financial resources 129
5.2.3 Impacts on physical and natural assets 131
5.2.4 HIV/AIDS impacts on livelihood activities 131
5.3 Social and moral aspects of HIV/AIDS impacts on the household 133
5.3.1 Family-based care 133
5.3.2 HIV/AIDS stigma 134
5.3.3 Secrecy and witchcraft-induced illness 138
5.4 Effects of HIV/AIDS on household food security 139
5.4.1 Empirical statistical analysis 140
5.4.2 Qualitative analysis 144
5.5 AIDS and livelihood vulnerability 146
5.6 Discussion and conclusions 150

Chapter 6 Interpersonal social relations: the limits of kinship and friendship – *No (wo)man is an island* **155**
6.1 Kinship relations 155
6.2 Friends and neighbours 162
6.3 Patron-client relations 169
6.4 Trust at interpersonal level 172
6.5 Interpersonal relations and gender 174
6.6 Discussion and conclusion 175

Chapter 7 A community in distress: the role of community-level social capital **179**
7.1 Social groups and organizations: inclusion and exclusion 179
7.1.1 Formal groups in the study area 180
7.1.2 Bridging social capital 184
7.1.3 Non-governmental organizations 185
7.2 Participation in groups 186
7.3 Community solidarity 191
7.3.1 Helping with day-to-day problems 191
7.3.2 Community voluntary and compulsory contributions 193
7.3.3 HIV/AIDS community-based interventions 194
7.3.4 Comparison with another village 196
7.4 Trust in the community: myths on community solidarity 198
7.5 Conclusion: safety nets with holes? 198

Chapter 8 General conclusions and discussion **203**
8.1 Conclusions 203
8.1.1 Dual disaster: HIV/AIDS and livelihood crisis 203
8.1.2 Degeneration or regeneration of social capital in the face of HIV/AIDS? 205
8.1.3 Implications of changes in social capital for household livelihood vulnerability 208
8.1.4 Household responses to the changing social capital and increased livelihood insecurity 209
8.2 Theoretical and methodological implications of the research 210
8.2.1 Social capital 210
8.2.2 Revisiting the household as a unit of analysis 213
8.2.3 Methodological notes 215
8.3 Implications for policies and interventions 216

References **219**

Appendix 1. Factors influencing household food security (N = 180) **239**

Summary **241**

About the author **245**

List of acronyms

AFREDA	Action for Relief and Development Assistance
AIDS	Acquired Immunodeficiency Syndrome
ANC	Antenatal clinic
ARV	Antiretroviral
AWLAE	African Women Leaders in Agriculture and Environment
BSc	Bachelor of Science
CBOs	Community Based Organisations
CCM	Chama Cha Mapinduzi
CD_4	Cluster of differentiation 4
CRDB	Cooperative Rural Development Bank
CUF	Civil United Front
DFID	Department for International Development
DGIS	Directorate General for International Cooperation
ESRF	Economic and Social Research Foundation
FANR	Food, Agriculture and Natural Resources
FAO	Food and Agricultural Organisation
FCND	Food Consumption and Nutrition Division
FGD	Focus Group Discussion
GDP	Gross Domestic Product
GNP	Gross National Product
Ha	Hectares
HIV	Human Immunodeficiency Virus
ICF	International Christian Fellowship
ICRW	International Center for Research on Women
IDS	Institute of Development Studies
IFAD	International Fund for Agricultural Development
IFPRI	International Food Policy Research Institute
K_1	Kilombero 1
K_2	Kilombero 2
KAP	Knowledge, Attitude and Practice
KCGA	Kilombero Cane Grower Association
MCH	Mother and Child Health
MEMKWA	Mpango wa Elimu Maalumu kwa watoto waliokosa
MFUMAKI	Mfuko wa Maendeleo Kidatu
MOA	Ministry Of Agriculture
MOH	Ministry of Health
MSc	Masters of Science
MVIWATA	Mtandao wa Vikundi vya Wakulima Tanzania
NACP	National AIDS Control Programme

NBS	National Bureau of Statistics
NGO	Non-Governmental Organisation
NMSF	National Multi Sectoral Strategic Framework
PhD	Doctor of Philosophy
PLWA	Persons Living With AIDS
PLWHA	Persons Living With HIV/AIDS
PMTCT	Prevention of Mother to Child Transmission
REPOA	Research on Poverty Alleviation
ROSCA	Rotating Saving and Credit Association
SACCO	Saving and Credit Cooperative
SADC	Southern African Development Community
SHDEPHA	Service Health and Development for People living positively with HIV/ AIDS
STI	Sexually Transmitted Infection
SUDECO	Sugar Development Corporation
TACAIDS	Tanzania Commission for AIDS
TANESCO	Tanzania Electrical Supply Company
TAZARA	Tanzania and Zambia Railways
TBC	Tuberculosis
TBA	Traditional Birth Attendant
TShs	Tanzanian Shillings
UKONS	United Kingdom Office of National statistics
UNAIDS	United Nations Program on HIV/AIDS
UNDP	United Nations Development Program
UNICEF	United Nations Children Education Fund
UNRISD	United Nations Research Institute for Social Development
URT	United Republic of Tanzania
USA	United States of America
UTAKE	Uganda, Tanzania and Kenya
UWT	Umoja wa Wanawake Tanzania
VCT	Voluntary Counseling and Testing
VEO	Village Executive Officer
WHO	World Health Organization

Glossary

Balozi	Ten-cell leader
Bibi	Grandmother
Jumbe	A leader of a group of people
Kazi ya kujitolea	Voluntary work
Kaya	Household
Kitenge	Is a piece of cloth that is decorated with a variety of colours and patterns; it is often worn by women around the chest or waist, over the head as a headscarf or as a baby-sling.
Kunyolewa	To be shaved
Masika	Rainy season
Mdudu	Insect
Mizimu	Ancestors
Mraba	Estimated 10 x10 foot steps piece of land
Muathirika	HIV/AIDS afflicted
Ndundame	Shaving specialist assistant
Nguto	Request to jokers to coordinate funeral activities
Nyumba kumi	Ten households in a neighbourhood
Nyasika	Staying with one's daughter as a temporal spouse
Sanda	Burial garment
Ugali	Meal made of maize flour
Ugonjwa wa kisasa	'Modern' sickness
Umeme	Electrical shock
Upatu	Informal saving and credit arrangement
Utani	Joking relationship
Vijiji vy ujamaa	Ujamaa villages
Watani	Jokers

Chapter 1

Introduction

1.1 Motivation for the study

The motivation to pursue this study stems from observations in rural settings where I had been working for eight years in development projects and in programs with men and women groups in the regions of Morogoro and Dodoma in Tanzania. I realized that among other problems troubling group performance and activities were HIV/AIDS-induced deaths and prolonged illnesses among group members and their relatives. I developed an interest in assessing how such networks and groups are being affected by HIV/AIDS, and how this ultimately impinges on rural livelihoods. Social networks and community groups are usually used as entry points to many development initiatives. In such groups and networks, people constantly interact, exchange, mutually influence, enable or constrain one another, and mobilize relationships with other people who might give access to resources and support in times of need. Social networks and personal relationships are important when support, survival, and social security are at stake. Where people share a sense of identity, hold similar values, trust each other and reciprocally do things for each other, there can be a positive impact on the social, political and economic components of the society they are living in. Social networks that provide access to resources and social support in this study are referred to as social capital. There are numerous examples demonstrating that social networks in the community, including those of relatives, neighbours and friends, but also formal groups such as voluntary associations, contribute to the well-being of those involved. Because of the importance of these social networks for rural household livelihood, I was compelled to conduct a thorough and comprehensive social capital assessment in rural communities in the face of HIV/AIDS. Congruent with a broader AWLAE[1] program on 'Enhancing the role of women in food systems in Africa', it was possible to undertake this study.

1.2 HIV/AIDS situation in the country

It was estimated that by the end of 2006, 42 million people in the world were living with HIV/AIDS. Sub-Saharan Africa is the region of the world that is most affected by the pandemic. An estimated 25 million people are living with HIV, and approximately

[1] AWLAE programs prepare women professionals in agriculture and the environment for leadership positions, thus enabling them to contribute in the formulation of policies that take women's concerns into account. These policies are expected to influence changes in the way men and women relate in all spheres of life.

3 million new infections occurred in 2006, and the pandemic has claimed the lives of an estimated 2.1 million people in this region. In the region around 2 million children under 15 are living with HIV and more than twelve million children have been orphaned by AIDS (UNAIDS & WHO, 2006). The HIV/AIDS pandemic has emerged as a developmental problem, having consequences going far beyond the health sector. Indeed, it has become a major crisis in many of the developing countries and in the absence of a cure or vaccine, the devastating impacts of the epidemic are far-reaching.

Tanzania as one of the sub-Saharan countries and among the poorest countries in the world is badly affected. The country is located in East Africa and covers an area of 945,000 square kilometers. Administratively, the country has 25 regions (20 in the mainland and 5 in the island of Zanzibar). The estimated population by 2003 was 34.5 million people with about 80 percent living in rural areas (URT, 2003a). About 36 percent of the population is living below the basic needs poverty line (URT, 2002) with an estimated per capital income of US$ 280 in 2005 (www.tanzania.go.tz accessed on 25/03/07). The spread of HIV/AIDS has significant effects, not only on the demographic composition of the country's population but also on social and economic structures. HIV infection is unevenly distributed across geographical areas, sex, age, and socio-economic classes. The average national HIV/AIDS prevalence rate is seven percent (TACAIDS, NBS & USAID, 2005). The epidemic has struck the most economically active group of adults aged 15-49, with women having higher prevalence rates (8%) than men (6%) (TACAIDS, NBS & USAID, 2005). Despite the continuous decline in prevalence rates since 2002, some districts are still having an infection rate of more than twenty percent. In rural Tanzania, the infection rate ranges between five and thirty percent (URT, 2005).

The national HIV/AIDS Surveillance Report shows that by the end of 2004, 1.9 million individuals in Tanzania were living with HIV (URT, 2005). It should be noted that these data are subject to underestimation because the National Aids Control Program (NACP) estimates that only one out of 14 cases are reported due to underutilization of health facilities, because many people are not willing to go for a HIV test and also because of delays in reporting. These figures may blur the true force of the epidemic, since HIV/AID impacts are not only felt by those affected, but indirectly affect a wider segment of the population. HIV/AIDS has led to a significant orphan population. As a consequence of AIDS mortality, UNAIDS & WHO (2006) estimated that by the end of 2006 there were about 1.1 million orphans in Tanzania. Because of HIV/AIDS the average Tanzanian life expectancy is 44 years as opposed to the projected 56 years without AIDS (World Bank, 2003). The predominant mode of HIV transmission is through heterosexual contacts accounting for over 90 percent of new AIDS cases, followed by mother-to-child transmission whereby the mother passes the HIV-virus to the child during pregnancy, at time of birth or through breastfeeding (TACAIDS, NBS & USAID, 2005). Another mode of transmission is through infusion of infected blood.

Age and sex specific prevalence of HIV shows that women are affected at a younger age than men. Women's prevalence is higher in the age bracket 20-39 years whereas for men prevalence is highest at 40-49 years of age (URT, 2005a). The clustering of cases in the age group 20-49 years suggest that the majority of the infection occurs in productive and reproductive active population. Of all AIDS cases reported in 2004, 55.6 percent were married (URT, 2005a). The Tanzania HIV/AIDS Indicator Survey 2003/04 shows that those who were in a marital union at the time of the survey had seven and eight percent prevalence rate for women and men respectively. Women in polygamous unions showed higher rates (10 %) of infection than married women who were not in polygamous marital union (7%) at the time of the survey (TACAIDS, NBS & USAID, 2005).

The HIV/AIDS Indicator Survey in Tanzania showed that the level of basic knowledge about HIV/AIDS has increased (TACAIDS, NBS & USAID, 2005). This study found that 87 percent of the women and 88 percent of the men indicate that the chances of getting HIV can be reduced by limiting sex to one partner who is not affected and who has no other partners. Seven in ten (69%) women and over six in ten men (63%) know that HIV can be transmitted from a mother to her child by breastfeeding. However, knowledge about antiretroviral drugs is far less widespread; only 17 percent of women and 19 percent of men know that there are special drugs to reduce the risk of mother to child transmission. Demonstrating the misconceptions about AIDS transmission, most people (82% women and 89% men) in the survey rejected the idea that HIV cannot be spread by witchcraft or other supernatural powers. However, these findings should not be interpreted as implying that those who report that HIV/AIDS can be transmitted by witchcraft do not know how it is transmitted. HIV/AIDS can be attributed to witchcraft as an excuse or denial of personal responsibility or as a way to cope emotionally with the disease.

Despite a widespread knowledge on HIV transmission and efforts to address and reduce stigma, in many parts of the country people living with HIV/AIDS are still seen as shameful and irresponsible. Such perceptions exemplify stigmatization, which may ultimately lead to the exclusion of affected individuals from the family and the wider community. Stigma is responsible for secrecy and denial, which hinder people from seeking counseling and testing for HIV. According to the Tanzania HIV/AIDS Indicator Survey report, only 15 percent of women and men interviewed had undertaken an HIV test before the survey (TACAIDS, NBS & USAID, 2005). Stigma attached to HIV/AIDS leads to community excuses as regards the responsibility of caring for and looking after those who are affected. Stigma is growing towards those who are affected. For instance, results from the Tanzania HIV/AIDS Indictor Survey show that fewer women (52%) than men (63%) would buy fresh vegetables from a shopkeeper if they know he or she is HIV positive. These data indicate that, in spite of rising awareness, knowledge gaps and misconceptions about HIV/AIDS persist. Unwillingness to buy from an affected individual could be linked to stigma as a result of ignorance (ICRW, 2002; 2003). One also has to be aware that peoples' knowledge, attitude and intended practice may be at odds with they actually do.

The HIV/AIDS epidemic spreads rapidly into rural areas. More than 10 percent of the women attending antenatal clinics in some rural areas were infected with HIV in 2003/04 (URT, 2005b). The growing rate of HIV/AIDS in rural areas is posing serious impediments to development processes, since more than 80 percent of the Tanzanian population is based in rural areas, contributing more than 50 percent to GDP and over 60 percent to export income. In the absence of an effective vaccine and insufficient treatment of opportunistic infections, the disease is usually fatal once one is affected (Bruce *et al.*, 2000), although there has been some development in Antiretroviral (ARV) therapy.

HIV/AIDS has been affecting people in different spheres of their lives. The increase of AIDS-related mortality is manifested through various effects such as a lower life expectancy, an increased economic dependency ratio, reduced productivity, increasing poverty and a growing number of orphans. Evidence from Makete (Tumushabe, 2005), Ulanga and Kilombero districts in Tanzania (ESRF, 2005) indicate that affected households in those districts are poorer than non-affected ones, and have responded to their adversity by adopting food-search behaviours that removes both adult and child labour from working on their own farms, thus leaving the affected households perpetually food insecure. Households fostering orphans have similar problems. HIV/AIDS is a serious threat in Tanzania as it contributes to poverty in many of the affected households. As in other sub-Saharan Africa countries, the stigma surrounding HIV/AIDS-affected individuals and households remains very strong. It therefore plays a major role in worsening HIV infection, obstructing care and support to affected members in the households and in the community.

1.3 Government responses to HIV/AIDS epidemic

HIV/AIDS was declared a national disaster in December 1999 and has been cited in the Tanzania Government Poverty Reduction Strategy Paper as one of the main impoverishing forces (URT, 2000). Therefore, reduction of the impact of the HIV/AIDS epidemic in Tanzania is identified as one of the strategies to reduce poverty (URT, 2000). HIV/AIDS is one of the government's highest priority development issues.

The country is making efforts to fight increased HIV transmission and its impacts. For almost two decades now, Tanzania has been undertaking various interventions to slow the spread of HIV infection and mitigate its effects. The National AIDS Control Program (NACP) was created in 1985 under the Ministry of Health, after which short and medium-term plans were formulated. Since HIV/AIDS impacts are not related to health alone, as its consequences stretch across different socio-economic spheres, there was a need for a multi-sectoral approach. Hence, in 2000 the Tanzania Commission for AIDS (TACAIDS) was established under the Prime Minister's office. Its mandate is to provide leadership and coordination of multi-sectoral responses. Further, the National Policy for HIV/AIDS was inaugurated in November 2001, and in May 2003 a National Multi-Sectoral Strategic Framework (NMSF) on HIV/AIDS 2003/07 was launched. NMSF translates the national HIV/AIDS policy by providing strategic guidance for the planning of programs, projects and interventions by various stakeholders in the fight against HIV/AIDS. The National Multi-Sectoral HIV/AIDS Strategic Framework states that the rate of HIV/AIDS infection and its impacts are to be reduced through a well-coordinated national response program that ensures comprehensive and effective community based HIV/AIDS interventions.

During the 1980s, the HIV/AIDS pandemic was believed to be largely concentrated in urban areas, townships and border posts, and was mainly associated with activities of truck drivers and prostitutes. As time went on, the disease spread into the general population and rural areas as a result of the growing links between rural and urban areas through for instance trade, farming opportunities, mining activities, rural-urban migration etc. Because of the spread of HIV/AIDS to rural areas, agriculture which is an important sector for the economy of the country and accounts for about 85 percent of the rural employment, is adversely affected. The effect of general poverty paired with high rate of HIV infection is dramatic, as the epidemic strikes at an already very vulnerable section of the population. The epidemic tends to worsen poverty and inequality because the low-income households are more adversely affected by AIDS deaths than other households. This situation has major implications for poverty alleviation and the welfare of the population.

Regardless of the efforts to curb HIV/AIDS effects in the country, it has been documented that current HIV/AIDS interventions in the country are mainly focusing on prevention and to a small extent on other thematic areas of intervention as specified in the National HIV/AIDS policy (ESRF, 2003). These include mitigation, care and support, and treatment. Little emphasis is being placed on the provision of these services. Access to ARV and treatment of AIDS-related infections is limited to a very small proportion of those in need. A lot is being done to increase community awareness, knowledge and condom provision. As stipulated in NMSF, community-based initiatives in collaboration with other stakeholders are very crucial actors in the fight against HIV/AIDS. Understanding local and associated factors is essential for obtaining an accurate appraisal of HIV/AIDS implications and properly prepares communities for the implementation of various interventions. Therefore, it is important to have a better understanding of how communities' informal and formal social networks operate in the face of HIV/AIDS and in the wider context in which community members interact.

1.4 Research problem and questions

The HIV/AIDS pandemic represents a great threat to food security and rural livelihoods. Morbidity and mortality due to HIV/AIDS affect household livelihood resources and assets, resulting in reduced ability of the household to generate livelihood and be prepared for future shocks. Households affected by HIV/AIDS suffer the loss of productive labour, income and food reserves. There is much evidence on the effects of HIV/AIDS on household's food insecurity. According to Barnett & Rugalema (2001), the combination of adult morbidity and mortality due to AIDS is associated with diversion and withdrawal of labour, which has led to a number of adverse changes in household food and livelihood security. Savings are diverted and assets are depleted to meet health care and funeral costs. More and more households and individuals are forced to seek support from the broader community. These mounting demands threaten existing social assets and long-standing local institutions. Since HIV/AIDS depletes a household's resources necessary for livelihoods, it may threaten the formation and maintenance of social networks that households need to mitigate HIV/AIDS impacts.

In some circumstances, a crisis such as prolonged sickness may result in strengthened social cohesion and may even generate new social relations that improve the overall social capital as poor communities find resourceful ways to overcome their problems (Robb, 1998). Several studies (Rugalema, 1999; Madembo, 1997; Topouzis & Hemrich, 1996, Lundberg *et al.,* 2000; Lwihula 1998; Mutangadura *et al.*, 1999) have indicated that households affected by HIV/AIDS get support primarily from the extended family, neighbours and community institutions as well as from the government. Gender and age are critical factors in accessing such support in the HIV/AIDS context (Bharat *et al,*. 2001; UNAIDS, 1999; Gillian, 1996; ICRW, 2003). Those affected by HIV/AIDS, especially women and orphans, face food shortage due to loss of productive resources, lack of assets caused by disinheritance, and exclusion from kinship and other social networks.

The preceding discussion shows that it is not fully clear how social capital produced in social networks is used, generated and maintained in the situation of HIV/AIDS. Some study results indicate that social capital is being eroded, while others report it being strengthened since new forms are emerging. This study argues that because of HIV/AIDS, social capital available to households is changing in form and content. Therefore, in order to understand the relationship between the AIDS impacts and rural livelihood security, it is necessary to relate analytically the changing nature of rural institutions and social networks to the changing rural livelihood within which food security is realized.

With regard to all these issues gender is a cross-cutting variable. HIV/AIDS impacts and susceptibility are gendered (Müller, 2005), and the same applies to access to the resources needed for generating livelihood. Women's disposal of and access to the various forms of social capital is generally known to be different from that of men (Molyneux, 2002). While such forms of social capital may indeed empower women, they also reflect the gendered nature of power relations between men and women. Household food security and care are important livelihood outcomes, and because of women's reproductive responsibilities their role in care giving and food procuring, processing, and preparing is generally far more important than that of men (Niehof, 2003). However, gender inequalities within the household often prevent women from enjoying the benefits of domestic production to the same degree as men. The advent of AIDS increases gender inequalities in access to resources as the epidemic reinforces the existing problems women face with regard to access and control over resources as well as in relation to care responsibilities.

This study intends to address the problem of the effects of HIV/AIDS on social capital, its implications for household vulnerability to food insecurity, and people's responses to these. The study was guided by the following hypotheses:

a) Households that are more vulnerable to HIV/AIDS impacts need more social capital to cope and mitigate these effects, yet they are not able to generate and maintain it.
b) Peoples' awareness of living in a HIV/AIDS-risk environment may give rise to new forms of collective responses.

From the research problem and hypotheses, four main clusters of questions were derived:

1. What are the direct effects of HIV/AIDS on household livelihoods?
2. What is the influence of HIV/AIDS on social capital?
3. What are the implications of changes in social capital for household livelihood vulnerability?
4. How do households respond to the changes in social capital and increasing livelihood insecurity?

1.5 Structure of the publication

This publication is organized in eight chapters. The conceptual and analytical framework is presented in Chapter 2 by means of a review of the relevant literature on households, livelihood, social capital, HIV/AIDS impacts and the relationship among them. Gender differentiation is taken into account throughout the discussion. Later, the linkages of concepts are shown in a figure depicting the conceptual framework.

Chapter 3 presents the research design and methods used in collecting empirical and secondary data. It describes different data sets and justifies the methods used to collect the data utilized in this study. It gives details on the sampling procedure and its limitations. Methodological discrepancies encountered and opportunities used to improve the quality and usefulness of the information gathered during the study, are also presented.

Chapter 4 provides details on the context in which the study was carried out. It offers a description of the study area including the history of the village. Livelihood activities and the role and effects of privatization of the Sugar Company in the area are presented and discussed. Basic social services, village social life, and the vulnerability context are also discussed.

Chapter 5 discusses gendered direct effects of HIV/AIDS in the households' livelihoods. These effects are through the household's resource base and activities portfolio and consequently in changes in the household's food security status. Social and moral aspects of HIV/AIDS impacts on individuals and households are discussed as well. Household responses to HIV/AIDS impacts are also presented.

Chapter 6 examines how interpersonal social ties play an important role in the management of HIV/AIDS effects and other day-to-day problems. HIV/AIDS impacts on interpersonal social relations are discussed, to see how they affect social relations and networks that influence people's livelihoods and their ability to respond to HIV/AIDS epidemic impacts and other shocks.

Chapter 7 specifically addresses HIV/AIDS impacts at the community level in a situation where there are other problems existing in the community. These were elicited by participation in formal networks and other collective activities in the community. Community characteristics such as presence of groups, NGOs, ethnic diversity, community programs, voluntary community contributions, and generalized trust which determine collective and the household's ability to cope with HIV/AIDS impacts are discussed. The chapter presents community responses to HIV/AIDS.

These are compared to those found in a neighbouring village and the differences are explained.

Chapter 8 presents a summary of the answers to the research questions. It also brings together findings from previous chapters and discusses their theoretical and practical implications. Policy and intervention recommendations are presented that might mitigate HIV/AIDS impacts and reduce household vulnerability.

Chapter 2

Household, livelihood, social capital and HIV/AIDS impacts: a conceptual and analytical framework

This chapter discusses the main concepts that are used in the formulation of the research problem and research questions. The discussion revolves around three core concepts: household, livelihood, and social capital, which are all gendered in nature. This chapter first reviews the theoretical discussion on the concepts and subsequently examines their interrelationships and importance for livelihoods outcomes such as food security, care, and coping. Concepts and the framework that depicts how HIV/AIDS is affecting different processes in the households and livelihood generation are discussed. In the literature review attention is paid to the way rural households are impacted by insecurities and how they deal with risks. Finally, it presents the linkages of important concepts in this study in the conceptual framework.

The household is important because it is the unit to which livelihood generation is anchored. It is the arena where much of daily life takes place and the centre of processes that determine the welfare of individual members. The household is the context in which members interact and pursue the activities to provide for their daily needs and well-being. As households' livelihood activities and strategies differ, they are at risk of different types of shocks. Shocks threaten household livelihoods or even their survival, which in turn increases household's vulnerability. A risky situation or shock may jeopardize a household's future livelihood. In such a situation a common response is to fall back on community-based social networks and family ties. Social networks between households of different kinds provide a sort of safety net for households that face various problems, which may prevent them from falling into poverty. Therefore social capital is an asset that can be used to diminish individuals and households' vulnerability to poverty and a means to sustain livelihoods. Although all households can be affected by stress and shocks, not all households are equally resilient. The extent to which households can make claims on social networks depends on their ability to build up their social capital.

This work builds on Rugalema's (1999a) work in Kagera in Tanzania. Rugalema focused on the processes and mechanisms through which morbidity and mortality consume household assets and lead to entitlement failure. His study reveals that prolonged adult morbidity and mortality due to AIDS have adverse effects on households primarily due to their effects on labour availability and depletion of other household resources. He confirms that illness and death affect time allocation, change household composition, put pressure on available labour, divert household cash, and lead to disposal of a household's productive assets. Changes imposed by AIDS on household endowments render survivors vulnerable. The study also found that because of AIDS the normal household cycle is disrupted, resulting in a variety of household types in terms of composition and headship, including households headed by orphans, the elderly and widows. Many of such households face difficulties in participating in both on and non-farm activities. Most of their productive activities are reduced because of loss of productive assets and partly due to the loss of labour. However, individuals and households are not passive; they actively explore ways to deal with the hardship brought about by AIDS. Rugalema shows how households relocate and transform their resources to cope with the losses induced by AIDS. The household's asset base and the gender and age of the survivors determine the household's ability to mitigate the effects of HIV/AIDS. Rugalema shows that HIV/AIDS affects livelihoods in a holistic manner and that its impacts are a process rather than a final outcome.

The impacts of HIV/AIDS are diverse and differ according to context. As the epidemic continues there is a need for more empirical research to improve the evidence base for designing appropriate interventions and policy-making. Therefore, there is a need to continuously assess how households are making their livelihoods as the context they are living in and the challenges they face are changing. Apart from the fact that the current study was carried out in a different area in Tanzania than Rugalema's study, it also has a different emphasis. It intends to investigate the impacts of HIV/AIDS on social resources accrued by participation in social networks characterized by reciprocity and trust.

Social networks are assumed to facilitate individuals and households to access resources but are also crucial for coping with the difficulties imposed by AIDS and other crises. This study moves beyond households by trying to show the connections between HIV/AIDS-affected and non-affected households by treating these connections as one of the resources those households deploy to cope with HIV/AIDS impacts. The study tries to fill in the gap by critically investigating the effects of HIV/AIDS on social networks and the trust invested in those networks that facilitate or impede peoples' recourse to social networks in times of AIDS. The study also explores impacts and response mechanisms raised at the collective level of the community. However, being aware that social networks do not operate in isolation from other resources the study investigates impacts of HIV/AIDS on social networks in relation to other resources.

2.1 Household

In this study the household is taken as the unit of analysis because it is the locus where resources are generated, organized, managed and used for economic activities as well as for the welfare of household members and care (Niehof, 2002; 2004b; 2004c). Most of these activities aim at fulfilling primary and daily needs of the household members, such as food, shelter, clothing, health and security. At the same time, it is recognized that households are embedded in and surrounded by support networks, notably kinship networks, friends, and neighbours. Conventionally, households are conceived of as a social group of which the members reside in the same place, share meals and make joint or coordinated decisions over resources allocation and income pooling. This definition places the emphasis on co-residence as the key attribute of the household (Ellis, 2000). However, due to increased rural livelihood diversification, migration has become a very common phenomenon leading to situations where household members are not always permanently in residence but may be spread over many different locations. The criterion of co-residence has to be interpreted in terms of proximity in a situation where members of a household are spread over different dwelling units in a single compound (Mtshali, 2002).

According to Rudie (1995:228) a household is a co-residential unit that is usually family-based and jointly manages resources to provide for its members' primary needs. In African countries, a household may comprise several houses, which belong to one family (Guyer & Peters, 1988). In this case there might be more than one 'cooking pot', which offers another way of classifying households (Fapohunda, 1988). Rudie's definition of household will be used in this study because it addresses dimensions of household that are relevant in this study: first, the dimension of resource management for household members' primary daily needs, and, second, co-residence which is glossed here as geographical proximity. For a household to be able to provide for its members on a daily basis, proximity is very important. Still non-resident household members may supply households with remittances, which are used to access food, labour and other needs, hence playing a role in family subsistence and maintenance. Even if non-resident members do not participate in the daily processes in the household, they may have decision-making responsibilities. Although to some extent decisions become freed from pre-established ties, in extended family and kinship structures relatives outside the household frequently still play an important role in decision-making (Omari, 1995). In this study, non-resident members are considered important for the household processes as a resource or a support relation to the household. They could be affiliated members and have to be distinguished from ordinary household members.

Households do not exist as discrete social and economic units but are connected to others in overlapping relationships. Because of this, Drinkwater (2003) proposed to use another analytical unit: the cluster. A 'cluster' is defined as a group of producers between whom multiple resource exchanges, usually based on kinship, labour, and possibly common access to resources, are taking place. A cluster can consist of various households, usually, though not necessarily, living in the same geographical area. Cluster analysis moves away from households as the unit of analysis to look at clusters of individuals and households, to make visible the complexity and fluidity of people's lives (Drinkwater, 2003; Drinkwater *et al.*, 2006). In times of HIV/AIDS, cluster analysis may help to explain how households adapt or disintegrate because of ill-health of their members. Another merit of the concept is that it allows an identification and understanding of important overlapping social relationships between individuals of different generations and gender, in relation to marital and kinship ties. It is argued that vulnerability in terms of gender, age, and socio-economic status, can only be understood clearly in the context of multiple resource flows and relationships among households. Nevertheless, this study used the household as the unit of analysis, though a unit with permeable boundaries (Guyer & Peters, 1988). Within the household individuals also have different positions based on gender and age that are reflected in patterns of authority and in the division and control of labour and other resources.

2.1.1 Intra-household differentiation

Internal differentiation and stratification of households are revealed in the diversity of activities and tasks individual members perform, and in the ways in which goods and services are distributed. Neo-classical models characterize households as unified production and consumption units in which labour is allocated according to principles of comparative advantages, income is pooled and preferences for consumption and leisure are shared. It is assumed that the authoritative male household head makes the decisions more or less to the benefit of all and that members profit equally from the household income. This view underestimates intra-household differences in terms of preferences, access to and control over resources, power in decision-making, and even in access to basic domestic services (Kabeer, 1991; O'Laughlin, 1995). In order to be able to capture and understand the relations of production and exchange within households, households should be viewed as differentiated units. According to Agarwal (1997) households comprise multiple actors with varying and often conflicting preferences and interests, and differential abilities to pursue and realize their interests. Households are seen as units that are not homogeneous; they differ in composition according to gender and age. Women and men have different control over resources, perform different economic activities, contribute differently to the household economy, and, hence, are likely to engage in different social networks (Boserup, 1970; 1998). The weakness of the neo-classic household model lies not only in its failure to deal with the individuals that make up the household, but also in its failure to recognize systematic gender and age-based power relations which structure household resource allocation (Katz, 1997). The household is one of the key institutional sites of gender inequality. The feminist critique of the unitary household model calls for specification of the gender of household members and the recognition that gender makes a difference in decision-making and allocation of resources.

Sen's (1990) model of the household as a domain of cooperative conflict is characterized by bargaining processes among the members of a household. Cooperation between different members allows them to achieve gains, which are unlikely to have accrued to any individual member acting on his or her own. However, conflict may arise about how the gains of cooperation are to be distributed. In many cases cooperation outcomes are more favourable to one party than the other, hence the underlying tension and conflict between the parties involved. Therefore, cooperation will depend on the relative bargaining power of the household member. This model of the household has an advantage over the classical unitary model because it recognizes the existence of more than one decision-maker within the household and the potential for conflicting objectives and strategies (Kabeer, 1991).

Although every individual in the household may have different strategies to get the best outcomes, to some extent there has to be a common strategy for the household to enable members to work towards achieving a common goal. Organization and management of household activity are important for the provision of day-to-day needs, and this has to involve some common understanding between the people living in the household. Households develop sets of governing rules of what is or is not acceptable behaviour by members and an understanding about household membership and access to properties and rights within the household. They develop working practices about the allocation of tasks or bringing in resources necessary to maintain the household. Such rules emerge through social interaction and have the character of an emergent property (Anderson *et al.*, 1994), which does not belong to any one member of the household. Hence, the household can have strategies which are more than the sum of the individual aspirations of its members. However, it should not be assumed that a household strategy is always based upon consensus. More often than not it is the result of negotiation and compliance.

Decision-making is considered to be a crucial process underlying all functions of the household resource management. It has been a central issue in gender relations discussions. Since the household has been subsumed under a joint unitary model, the issue of power among household members is not explained; hence the differences among members do not come to the fore. Also the assumption that decisions are based on rational choice results in the reductionist view of the reality of a household's everyday life (Pennartz & Niehof, 1999). Decision-making in the household involves tension between the welfare of the collective and the needs and desires of the individuals. In the event of a shock like HIV/AIDS, conflicts of interest may be intensified and can push individual household members to the point where they refuse to cooperate.

The decision-making process is influenced by the bargaining power of the parties involved. Both Kabeer (2003) and Agarwal (1997) mention men's and women's separate spheres of decision-making based on socially recognized gender roles, while sharing some common responsibilities and some resources and activities. Those decisions related to daily household maintenance in terms of food are made by women, while those with more far-reaching consequences for the household and family are often made by men. An individual's position with regard to gender and generation is an important factor in decision-making processes in Africa (Armstrong, 1997). Decision-making also relates to power. Power and authority is vested in the member who has control over the general affairs of the household unit, including decision-making concerning its economic, social and political affairs (Bookwalters and Warner, 2001). Through gender-based frameworks and gendered privileges, men are legitimized to hold more decision-making power. In Tanzania, as in many other African societies, patrilineal kinship and patriarchy characterize power invested in men rather than women and influence decision-making in favour of men. Traditionally, the oldest man in the household occupies the position as the nominally dominant person with well-defined rights over other household members, having authority over decisions on household property and assets. In patrilineal societies, where decision-making is skewed in favour of men, women's needs and preferences are easily glossed over. This has great implications for women's ability to cope with HIV/AIDS impacts.

The position of men as key decision-makers is challenged when the relations between household members change and are renegotiated. Women are increasingly occupying a decision-making position. For example, the involvement of women in wage employment and in the informal sector has tilted power relations within the household (Koda, 1995). Participation of women in the labour market affects the allocation of their time for domestic chores and the contribution to the family income which has a bearing on their decision-making in the household. Migration, recent trends in mortality, and a growing number of women living in consensual unions as well as women having children prior to or outside marriage, have resulted in *de facto* female household headship. Women may also acquire *de jure* headship through marriage dissolution in the event of death, separation or divorce, though in some cases a widow will not assume household headship when a son is old enough to assume it.

2.1.2 Kinship and inter-household relations

Kinship and marriage form the basis of the family-based household. Members of a kinship network acquire the status of a relative by birth, marriage, or adoption. Generally, while blood relationship provides the basis for kinship, the way it is used and defined is determined by socio-cultural considerations (Howard, 1986; Harris, 1990). Kinship is much more than biologically determined relationships; not all people considered kin have blood ties. According to Harris (1990:31-32), 'the only thing kinship systems have in common is that they are cognitive systems employed for the ordering of social relationships which have reference to some aspect of 'physical' kinship'. In different societies the same biological relationship may be perceived differently. Kinship is a basic principle of social organization. It lies at the base of many political, economic and even religious organizations, and serves as a medium for transmitting status and property from one generation to the next through the process of inheritance. Kinship controls social relationships between people in a community, governs marital customs and, to a large extent, social interactions. It also regulates access to means of production such as land and other resources. Kinship can be investigated by looking at empirically found kinship practices and the meaning of these practices and kinship relationships for the actors (Niehof, 2003a).

One of the major problems with neo-classic household economics was its failure to recognize intra-household relations and the social embeddedness of households within wider social networks. Household arrangements are geared towards long-term stable relationships within which reproductive and productive activities are organized for daily as well as inter-generational reproduction (Kabeer, 1994). The stability of relationships within households reflect principles of kinship and residence by which members are bound to each other through socially sanctioned implicit contracts which spell out their claims and obligations to each other. Pennartz & Niehof (1999:206) view the household as a context of 'condensed morality', meaning that household and kinship provide an overlapping moral context within which people acknowledge obligations and rights to give and receive support. Physical proximity and sharing daily life reinforce people's moral commitments towards each other. Households are embedded in larger structures such as kinship networks and community organizations or even the state, and their boundaries are permeable (Guyer & Peters, 1988). In the Tanzanian context households are related to one another in a variety of ways, including kinship, marriage, neighbourhood, gender-based groups, village-wide clubs, markets, and even formal institutions through an array of rights and responsibilities, claims and obligations.

Kinship relationships are motivated by non-economic factors and such transactions and exchanges, though based on moral principles, have economic functions and implications. In African societies kinship serves as a primary organizing feature for the production of goods and services. People work together and exchange what they produce because they are kin, and they do so in accordance with behavioural expectations linked to kinship (Brown and Thakur, 1997). Kinship relations are sustained by clearly defined obligations attached to specific roles within kinship networks. Kinship and extended family structures compose a wide range of claims and obligations and are characterized by reciprocity and redistribution. To describe these aspects Cheal (1989) and Scott (1976) use the term moral economy. Scott used the term to characterize support relations in Southeast Asia peasant communities. Cheal narrowed it down to apply to the household. The concept implies that households or communities are essentially geared towards providing social and economic security for all their members.

Trust and commitment are important factors in the sustainable functioning of the moral economy. Sometimes an individual or household may commit resources to support vulnerable kin members, not because of expected reciprocity in the future but because of social norms. By these norms kin are supposed to be supportive and give other kin access to resources. There are always expectations that people will be there for their relatives. People have a normative claim on their relatives' help in dealing with difficulties and mobilizing collective support. Different from kinship networks, friendship networks are voluntary and function as separate ties outside kinship groups. Because of their voluntary nature people must maintain them more actively. Thus, people are more concerned about reciprocating a friend's help than a relative's help (Wellman & Wortley, 1989). This implies that reciprocity is an important mechanism for the maintenance of friendships by defining the responsibility for each other. Friendship networks can be effective in handling immediate day-to-day problems.

In Tanzania all those who trace their origin back to a common ancestor belong to the same kin group, the members of which have a special relationship. There are both patrilineal and matrilineal groups. The distribution of authority and power in kinship groups has implications for people's access to resources. In a patrilineal society, the inheritance rights are given to the men. Generally, women are discriminated against with regard to inheritance rights. This has a serious effect on women's ability to access and control productive resources for sustaining the livelihoods of their families when their husbands fall ill or die of AIDS. Kinship institutions are also sites for the reproduction and transmission of patriarchal relations within society. Evidence suggests that they may be the site of mistrust, conflict, and deception, and may stifle women's freedom of speech and their ability to exercise individual choice (Dikito-Wachtmeister, 2001). In some societies, husbands can refuse their wives permission to occupy decision-making positions or attend decision-making meetings. In these situations, family and kinship ties are not necessarily beneficial to women, but may actually constrain women's ability to develop their own networks and benefit from them.

There has been an observable reduced reliance of households on kin in some societies. Such changes may be attributed to the development of capitalism, which gives rise to nuclear families, privatization of land and the strengthening of monetary values (Ottosson, 1999). For people who have been marginalized by the market economy, kinship continues to be of considerable significance by providing a source of security (Baerends, 1994). Therefore, changes in kinship relations are going to be to their disadvantage. Because in kinship moral obligations are involved, it is important for care giving both within households and beyond. This is very important in the face of HIV/AIDS, where the kinship networks have a responsibility in caring for AIDS patients and assist the surviving members of the affected household.

In summary, the household in the context of this study is defined as a group of individuals, not necessarily all linked by kinship ties, who live together and share the daily functions to provide for their basic needs. Household members vary according to sex and age as well as according to access and control over resources, including social resources. These variations within the household may influence the possibilities of household members to engage in social networks. The household is considered an arena of potential conflict because of these variations, but at the same time it provides the context of cooperation based on trust and shared values, which form the basis of joint household strategies. Cooperation is very important when it comes to coping with the consequences of HIV/AIDS. For instance, morbidity and mortality due to HIV/AIDS affect the time use of healthy members and influence household decisions regarding the allocation of resources within the household that are needed for their livelihoods and to cope with the impacts AIDS. The household's ability to solicit resources by virtue of its membership in various social networks of relatives, neighbours, and friends is important in coping with social exigencies. This implies that households are not isolated units but maintain linkages with the wider society. Relations beyond the household are an important source of social support for most rural households. These relationships are important when studying the impact of HIV/AIDS on households in rural communities because it is where an affected household might get support to cope with its impacts and deal with other adversities.

2.2 The livelihood framework

A livelihood concerns the way people shape their lives by using material and non-material assets (Kaag *et al.* 2004). It includes activities that people undertake to provide for their basic needs. The most common definition of livelihood was given by Chambers & Conway (1992:6) as:

> *'Capabilities, assets (store, resource, claim and access) and activities required for a means of living: a livelihood is sustainable if it can cope with and recover from stress and shock, maintain or enhance its capabilities and assets, and provide a sustainable livelihood opportunities for the next generation; and which contributes net benefits to other livelihoods at the local and global levels and in the short and long run.'*

The livelihood framework is a tool to help understand the livelihoods of the poor (Ellis, 2000). The framework is generally people-centred, holistic and focuses on the multi-dimensionality of daily life (Kaag *et al.*, 2004). The core of the livelihood approach lies in its analysis of the different assets or capital endowments upon which individuals or households draw to produce livelihood outcomes. The five groups of assets that are combined in different ways to generate livelihood outcomes include:

- Natural capital: the natural resource reserves from which resources useful for livelihoods are derived (e.g. land, water, wildlife, biodiversity, and environmental resources).
- Human capital: the skills, knowledge, ability to labour and good health important to the ability to pursue different livelihood activities.
- Physical capital: the basic infrastructure (transport, shelter, energy and communications) and the physical equipment and means that enable people to pursue their livelihoods.
- Social capital: the social resources (networks, membership of groups, relationships of trust, access to wider institutions of society) upon which people draw in pursuit of livelihoods.
- Financial capital: financial resources which are available to people (whether savings, suppliers of credit or regular remittances or pensions) and which provide them with different livelihood options.

The five livelihood assets in the sustainable livelihood framework are moulded by policies, processes and institutions to give desirable outcomes, such as more income, improved food security and reduced vulnerability. If achieved, these desirable outcomes then feed back to help build the capital asset base. Undesirable outcomes, such as increased vulnerability or a less supportive and cohesive social environment, erode the asset base. Policies, institutions, and processes affect how people use their assets in pursuit of different livelihood strategies. These refer to both formal and informal institutions and organizations that shape livelihoods by influencing access to assets, livelihood strategies and vulnerability. The vulnerability context (seasonality, shocks and trends) impacts on people's assets and options available to them. On the other hand, the vulnerability context can bring about new developments such as technological innovations. Threats that affect vulnerability can include periodic droughts, floods, pest infestations, economic shocks, crop and livestock shocks, conflict and civil unrest, as well as the illness and death. By utilizing different assets, individuals and households adjust to their physical, social, economic and political environments through a set of livelihood strategies designed to strengthen their well-being. Chambers (1989:6) describes livelihood sustainability as the ability to maintain and improve livelihoods while maintaining or enhancing the assets and capabilities on which livelihood depend. An individual's or group's livelihood is sustainable if it can adequately satisfy self-defined basic needs and is secure against shocks and stresses (De Haan, 2000). Household livelihood security is defined as a situation of adequate and sustainable access to income and resources to meet basic needs, including access to food, potable water, health facilities, educational opportunities, housing, time for community participation and social integration (Frankenberger & McCaston, 1998). Depending on the quality of livelihood outcomes some livelihoods are better than others and they can differ in their degree of sustainability or vulnerability (Niehof & Price, 2001).

Rural households engage in multiple activities and rely on diversified income portfolios for their livelihoods. In Tanzania for the past two decades there has been a process going on that Bryceson (1997) designates as 'de-agrarianisation', which refers to the process by which the population is becoming less agrarian in nature year by year. Although agriculture is still the main activity in rural areas, households increasingly pursue off-farm and non-farm activities for their livelihood. This is what Ellis (2000:15) calls livelihood diversification. He defines it as 'the process by which rural families construct a diverse portfolio of activities and social support capabilities in their struggle for survival in order to improve their standard of living'. He points out that diversification as a livelihood strategy is reflected in the varied nature of the livelihood portfolio. Rural people diversify their livelihood portfolio by getting involved in income generating activities such as petty trade, wage labour, handicraft, and brewing, and providing services such as tailoring, hairdressing/cutting, traditional medical care, etc. Engagement in a diverse portfolio of activities also entails nurturing the social networks of kin and community that enables such diversity to be sustained.

Livelihood diversification may be associated with success at achieving livelihood security under improving economic conditions and with livelihood distress in deteriorating conditions (Ellis, 2000, 1998; Niehof, 2004a). In the latter case, diversification is treated as a deliberate household strategy of making ends meet in the event such as floods, drought, and illness (Bryceson, 1997). Therefore, livelihood diversification may occur as a coping or an adaptive strategy. Through diversification of income households may reduce risks and achieve goals of enough income for livelihood security (Bryceson, 1997). An increase in different activities in rural areas has resulted in various changes in the agricultural economy and social relations among household members as well as in lifestyles of rural households. Migration and off-farm employment affect the organization of labour within households. As rural people become more mobile, the division of labour by gender changes, with women assuming more responsibilities for managing farms and domestic work (Berry, 1993). In Africa today there is a noticeable trend towards what has been termed 'feminization of agriculture'. As men's participation in agriculture declines, the role of women in agricultural production becomes more dominant (Price & Brouns, 1999; FAO, 1995). War, sickness and death from HIV/AIDS as well as migration of men from rural areas to towns and cities in search of paid employment have reduced rural male populations. For instance, in southern Africa where the HIV/AIDS pandemic is quite serious, male adult mortality levels for those who are in their productive years (15-59) range from 57 percent in South Africa to 72 percent in Zambia (Ngom & Clark, 2003). Problems associated with HIV/AIDS morbidity and mortality limit meeting basic needs such as those of food and care.

2.2.1 Household production of care

The household represents 'the arena of everyday life' for the majority of people (Clay & Schwartzweller, 1991). It is within this unit that many activities to provide for people's basic needs are undertaken. The care giving to the young, sick, disabled, and old members is part of the function of the household. Care is especially important to the sick and orphaned in times of HIV/AIDS because of the prolonged nature of illness and ensuing dependence. Tronto (1993:103) defines care as 'a species activity that includes everything that we do to maintain, continue and repair our 'world' so that we can live in it as well as possible. The world includes our bodies, ourselves, and our environment, all of which we seek to interweave in a complex, life sustaining web'. Tronto regards care as a one of the central activities in human life. Her definition is very broad, but Tronto stipulates that for an activity to be called care it has to include both care practices and the intention to care. She defines care as practice and places it in an overall social context.

To describe the quality of care Tronto (1993) proposes a new paradigm that centres on the ethics of care. Tronto sees care as having four separate but interconnected phases:

- *Caring about*: The recognition that care is necessary, which requires attentiveness.
- *Taking care of*: Assuming responsibility for the identified needs which also requires agency
- *Care-giving*: The direct meeting of the needs of care involving physical work and face-to-face contact. To do this one requires competence.
- *Care-receiving*: the response to the care received and its adequacy.

Tronto adds a fifth aspect: the integration of all four phases into a well-integrated care process. Her framework is useful in analyzing and judging the adequacy of care provided by the household as well as state institutions. The exchange of goods and services within the household is based on principles of reciprocity and morality (Cheal, 1989; Pennartz & Niehof, 1999). For example, support to dependent and weak members of the household is based on moral obligations.

Based on Tronto's conceptualization of care, competencies and resources are needed to provide adequate care (Niehof, 2004b). Both tangible and intangible resources are necessary for the household production of care. However, due to the intra-household division of labour, differential access to and control over resources and unequal decision-making power, availability of resources alone does not guarantee adequate care for all household members. Care processes are gendered in nature. In many societies women dominate the 'care-giving' phase, while the 'taking care of' phase is usually dominated by people with authority and control over resources who are mostly men. This shows that women and men play different roles in care processes, according to societal norms and values about gender. Care-giving within the household is part of domestic labour (Tronto, 1993; Luxton, 1997), which is unpaid and is carried out for the benefit of other household members. The primary responsibility for this is usually allocated to women. However, due to inequitable relationships within the household, women who are traditionally the care-givers may be denied the resources needed for care-giving. Lack of access to resources affects women's capability to provide care and satisfy the basic needs for their family's survival.

Because households are not isolated units, members from one household may have commitments and obligations to provide domestic labour for members in other households like those of relatives and friends. When the care needs exceed what the household can provide, the household may turn to its external network of relatives and friends, or to the state (Niehof, 2004b). In highly HIV/AIDS-affected countries, support from outside the households is decreasing while care needs are increasing, due to effects of AIDS and economic hardships. As a consequence of HIV/AIDS impacts, affected households lack the necessary resources to provide care and other basic necessities. Food provision to household members is an important aspect of care.

2.2.2 Household food security and its determinants

Food security is a basic need in human life and an important element of sustainable livelihood (Niehof & Price, 2001). According to the sustainable livelihood approach, food security is not just an issue of productivity but is about how people, especially poor people, gain access to production and can exchange capabilities in order to get food (Swift & Hamilton, 2001). Food security is the most critical indicator of livelihood insecurity. Yet it is difficult to discuss food security independently of wider livelihood considerations. Food security is defined as access by all people at all time to enough food for an active and healthy life (World Bank, 1986; FAO, 1997). This definition touches on many aspects:

Aspect	Implication
All people	Equity
At all times	Stability of food availability, access and utilization throughout the year and over time. Protection against risks affecting food availability.
Access to	Having the entitlements and means to access food through own production (landownership), purchase (affordability, purchasing power, food market prices), or gifts (social entitlements) of food.
Enough food	Enough food to meet the daily food requirements, sufficient stocks at household and community-level to resist shocks.
For an active and healthy life	Nutritious, safe, and culturally appropriate foods. Proper consumption and a good biological utilization of food resulting in an adequate health status.

The current definition of food security stipulates not only access by all people at all times to enough food for an active and healthy life, but includes access to secure sustainable livelihoods (Anderson & Cook, 1999). Historically, food security has been considered in terms of overall regional, national or even global food supplies and shortfalls in supply compared to requirements (Maxwell, 1996). A number of researchers have observed that there is an increased disparity in the sufficiency of food intake by certain groups, despite overall adequacy of supply (Sen, 1981; URT/MOA, 1997; Omosa, 1998). Therefore, instead of focusing on food supply only, the concept of food security has been broadened to include elements of access, vulnerability and sustainability. It has also evolved from focusing on food availability to a focus on food utilization and adequacy, which relates food to nutrition at individual level. The predominant way of thinking about food security has changed considerably over time. It has changed to become more holistic in nature, complex and people-centred.

This food security paradigm shift was brought about by the work of Amartya Sen. His famous book (1981) specifies that food flows stem from one's entitlements. A family's or person's ability to command subsistence goods (including food) and services depends on endowments (what a person owns as assets, labour, power, capital) and also on exchange entitlement mapping (the exchange possibilities) that exist through production and trade, which determine the consumption set available to a person with given endowments. Therefore, food insecurity became foremost a problem of 'access', even in famine situations. At issue here is not absolute availability of food, but the ability of the households to afford what is or could be available. The entitlement framework proved to be a powerful tool in understanding food insecurity in various circumstances and populations (Maxwell, 2001; Swift, 1989; Devereux, 1993). However, in the entitlement framework, the contribution of non-market food transfers through social networks and structures has been overlooked (Adams, 1993).

In their technical review on household food security, Maxwell & Frankenberger (1992) urge that a household is the logical unit for assessing food security because this is where decisions regarding food production and consumption are made. Food security is not only about food production through agriculture. It is, fundamentally, about incomes and distribution of resources and the way in which people use these resources to feed themselves. Food availability at the household level is achieved by own-production, purchases, gathering or donation/exchanges. Within households, women play a key role in ensuring food security because it is part of their reproductive role (Niehof, 2003). In food production, handling and preparation women play a significant role. To perform these tasks it is necessary that they have the means. According to Kavishe & Mushi (1993) and Baerends (1994), women have limited access to and control over means of food production and also insufficient purchasing power to access food. This has a direct and detrimental effect on their ability to guarantee household food security.

Food security is an important outcome of rural livelihood generation and in this study is used as a poverty indicator. The study addresses the concept of food security in terms of availability and access aspects. Food security in this study is defined as adequate access to food at all times throughout the year. Access to food can be achieved through own production and through the ability of households to generate sufficient income to meet food needs. Food security is examined by considering intra-household variations based on gender and age. Since there are multiple and varied sources of food security, which in most cases are not recorded or measured, it is difficult to make a complete analysis of household food security. Therefore, coping behaviours that households adopted were used as proxies for their food security status. These included changes in menu and meal patterns, sale of assets for food, and getting assistance from outside the household. The severity of the application of these behaviours gave an indication of the household food insecurity level. Other indicators include experiences with food shortage, access to remittances, amount of food stocks, involvement in income generation, and also the number and type of assets that a household owns.

2.2.3 Livelihood vulnerability

Livelihoods encompass crucial issues such as sustainability, vulnerability and coping. Vulnerability analysis has its roots in the political economy analyses of causes and consequences of drought and famine articulated between 1970 and 1980. Many studies on vulnerability draw upon Sen's concept of endowments, entitlement and rights, linking the local experiences of vulnerability to the broader institutional structures that reproduce it, as well as to opportunities for social action to alter it (Sen, 1990, quoted in Eakin, 2005). Although the concept of vulnerability has its roots in disaster studies, it refers to more general dynamics. It is embedded in complex power relations, resource distribution, knowledge and technological development. Vulnerability is not a predetermined state, but is socially constructed, contextual, dynamic and driven by various causes and processes. Changing social and environmental conditions such as urbanization and deforestation, for example, can influence vulnerability. Vulnerability is also often the result of interacting stresses and pressures in a given context. For example, the spread of HIV/AIDS is increasing vulnerability to global environmental change in sub-Saharan Africa by impacting the local labour force and reducing local adaptive capacities. The consequences of such multiple stresses are visible in some southern African countries that face severe drought and are being hardly hit by HIV/AIDS simultaneously (Vogel & O'Brien, 2004).

The words vulnerable and vulnerability are now common terms in the development discourse, but they are not always precisely used. Vulnerability tends to be used as a synonym for poverty but it is not the same (Moser, 1998). It is not always the poor that are the most vulnerable to environmental stress (Wisner *et al.*, 2004). Although poor households are among the most vulnerable because of resource constraints, rich households may also become vulnerable due to shocks such as natural disasters, economic shock and crisis, illness or death of the breadwinner. Poverty is about not having enough now, while vulnerability is the probability that one will fall into poverty in the future. Poverty is in most cases only measured at a single point in time and defined as shortfall in current income or expenditure. Vulnerability refers to a dynamic process implying that there is a chance that a currently non-poor may end up being poor in the future, whereas a currently poor person also has a chance to escape from poverty if there are changes in economic conditions resulting in an increase of income. Put simply, vulnerability is the probability that an individual, household or community will experience a decline in well-being in the future.

Moser (1996) notes that there is no widely accepted definition of vulnerability and its indicators. Various authors have defined it from different perspectives. Moser herself argues that vulnerability is caused by lack of assets and the way people are managing their assets in dealing with and recovering from disasters. She (1996:240) defines vulnerability as 'the well-being of individuals, households or communities in the face of changing environment'. Chambers (1989) refers to vulnerability as people's exposure to contingencies and stress and their difficulty in coping with them. Blaikie *et al.* (1994:9) define vulnerability as 'the characteristics of a person or group in terms of their capacity to anticipate, cope with, resist and recover from the impacts of natural hazard'. Ellis (2000) describes vulnerability as a household's inability to cope with adverse situations given its assets and resources. Devereux (2001) uses vulnerability as a concept that combines exposure to a threat with susceptibility or sensitivity to its adverse consequences. Christiaensen & Boisvert (2000) define vulnerability as the probability of living standards falling below some reference level in future. Wisner *et al.* (2004) define vulnerability as the characteristics of a person or group and their situation that influence their capacity to anticipate, cope with, resist and recover from the impact of natural hazards. Dercon (2005) describes vulnerability as an ex-ante situation, i.e. before one has knowledge of the actual shocks that will occur. Vulnerability also measures the resilience against risks. This is what is called adaptive capacity, defined here as those characteristics of an individual, household, or population group that enable those concerned to alter or structurally reorganize their activities to diminish present threats to survival while enhancing its ability to address new risks.

According to Winchester (1992) a household's characteristics also determine its level of vulnerability, notably the way people live, the assets and resources they share, and the nature of support networks, labour power and productivity as indicated by household size and composition. Households do not remain constant but change with time. As households make a transition from one life-course stage to another, resources undergo reallocation to accommodate the changes in household demand and circumstances. Households adapt to changing circumstances. Household changes over time have been analyzed by using a life-cycle model and, recently, a life-course model. Although these two models are used interchangeably, they differ conceptually. The life-cycle approach addresses the development stages and sequence of roles through which the individual passes from birth to death, whereas the life-course approach looks at alternative series of roles and experiences through which an individual passes from birth to death, and inquires into the causes and impacts of the variation in these patterns (Kertzer, 1986). The life-cycle approach assumes a typical progression through a given number of stages in more or less predetermined order (Murphy, 1987). Finch (1987) and Kertzer (1986) describe the life-cycle approach as being too static, while Pennartz & Niehof (1999) call it too normative. It would be appropriate if societies were unchanging, but there are various reasons why individuals or families may not conform to a typical life-cycle model. These may include death, marital breakdown, a decision not to get married or having children before marriage. The life-course approach focuses on the actual experience of individuals and the different pathways of households through the life course. The essence of the life-course approach lies in its focus on the continuous interplay between social, economic, cultural and political changes and the life course of an individual or a household. Hence, the concept of life course views life as a series of states, transitions, events and processes occurring in life (Berger *et al.*, 1996). Life-course dynamics highlight the issue of control. In case of a crises such as HIV/AIDS, households are faced with an involuntary break in the life course to the extent that household can no longer pursue the anticipated and desired life course (Pennartz & Niehof, 1999). Crises may cause households to loose control and render previous strategies inapplicable.

The household's composition reflects its stage in the household life course (Ali, 2005), which is is important in relation to the use of household resources and indicative of labour availability in the household. Based on her analysis in four communities Moser (1996) argue that household composition and stage in the life course are critical factors in determining household ability to cope with economic difficulties. Morbidity and mortality affect the household dependency ratio, which in turn affects livelihood strategies and outcomes. Young-adult AIDS mortality disrupts the household's life course. Rugalema (1999) showed that AIDS mortality affects the household life course and uses the household dependency ratio as an indicator for this.

Recognizing that vulnerability is contextual and social, Sen (2002) has viewed vulnerability from two different perspectives. The first perspective may be called the risks-centric view whereby vulnerability is typically defined as variability in living standards caused by consumption or income shocks. The second perspective may be called the rights-centric view whereby vulnerability is used to express the lack of social and political rights. Both are important in considering the implications of vulnerability for poverty. The first tends to highlight transient poverty, the second focuses on chronic poverty. However, most of the analysis in the current vulnerability literature is restricted to evidence on risks and shocks that generate variability in living standards and pay relatively little attention to the social, political and psychological aspects of vulnerability caused by powerlessness, lack of voice and lack of rights. Gender inequality is addressed in rights-centric view. This means that vulnerability is also manifested in the gender hierarchies in the community and women's experience of marginalization and discrimination.

Blaikie *et al.* (1994:48) acknowledge that vulnerability is structured by relations of gender and power intersecting at different institutional sites:

> *'Gender is a pervasive division affecting all societies, and it channels access to social and economic resources away from women and towards men. Women are often denied the right to vote, the right to inherit land, and generally have less control over income-earning opportunities and cash within their own households. Normally their access to resources is inferior to that of men. Since our argument is that less access to resources, in the absence of other compensations to provide safe conditions, leads to increased vulnerability, we contend that in general women are more vulnerable to hazard.'*

Gender relations within households perpetuate inequalities between men and women, thereby increasing women's vulnerability. Coupled with poverty that women have to deal with, they also face enormous disadvantages that are embedded in gender relations. While they often have poor access to intra-household resources and lack decision-making power, poor women are responsible for meeting the reproductive needs of the household and have to play a productive role as well. Gender biases in labour markets and social exclusion that women experience in a variety of economic and political institutions contribute to the greater vulnerability of women as compared to men. The concept of 'feminization of poverty' describes the increasing poverty among women which also highlights their vulnerability. Despite the fact that a lot of studies argue that women are generally more vulnerable than men, there is also contrasting evidence. In her study in South Africa, Mtshali (2002) found that there was no difference between female-headed and male-headed households in terms of wealth. She observed that women without husbands are under less patriarchal control than women in male-headed households, hence have more freedom of movement to pursue different activities. Nevertheless, Niehof (2004a) points to female household heads' insecurity due to lack of entitlements under legal and customary rights. Chant (2003) notes that there is a lack of fit between available macro and micro-level data and the claim that female-headed households are always poorer. Female headship is not always correlated to poverty (Appleton, 1996).

Vulnerability is a relative term. Within any community some members are likely to be more vulnerable than others. Although a community may face the same risks, members will not be equally vulnerable. Ability to avoid or reduce vulnerability depends not only on initial assets but also on the ability to transform them into income, food and other basic necessities (Moser, 1998). According to a World Bank report (2000b), a household or individual can become more vulnerable to poverty for several reasons: first, lack of physical assets to sell to compensate loss of income and, second, limited human capital in terms of education and labour. The third reason can be lack of a social insurance system provided by the government or an informal safety net provided by family or local community. Though having resources does not guarantee that households will effectively manage changing patterns of risks, they do provide them with the means to negotiate new risks as they arise and evolve (Eakin, 2005). As Bebbington (1999:2022) argues, 'assets are not simply resources; they are also the basis of agents' power to act and to reproduce, challenge or change the rules that govern the control, use and transformation of resources'. Vulnerability is determined by the options available to households and individuals to make a living, the risks they face and their ability to handle these. According to Ellis (2000) people diversify their livelihoods to prevent future vulnerability.

Livelihood studies differentiate between the internal and external side of vulnerability (Chambers, 1989). The contexts in which people live in constitute the external side of vulnerability. These are factors that are beyond individual's control but affect their livelihood, such as ecological changes, market trends, demographic changes, political turmoil, failing health infra-structures, and social inequality. The external dimension involves exposure to risks and shocks. According to Brons *et al.* (2007) external vulnerability is part of the societal or ecological context but influences individual vulnerability and coping behaviours. The internal side of vulnerability refers to the capacity to anticipate risk, cope with, resist and recover from the impacts of shocks, which relate to specific characteristics of the person or group who are exposed to these. These include characteristics of individuals (e.g. age, sex, health status, skills) and household characteristics (gender of household head, income, dependency ratio and assets-ownership). The internal dimension of vulnerability comprises lack of assets and entitlement failures. The extent to which individuals or groups are entitled to make use of resources determines their ability to cope with and adapt to stress (Sen, 1990). Table 2.1 shows different indicators of internal and external vulnerability as adapted and modified from Moser's (1996) framework.

Brons *et al.* (2007) argue that in order to understand poverty there is a need to look at external and internal vulnerability dimensions of household vulnerability and the individual and aggregate effects of people's activities to improve their livelihoods. External ecological and socio-economic dynamics have differential impacts on

Table 2.1. Vulnerability factors.

Source	Internal indicators	External indicators
Economic	Wage decline, job loss, property loss. Lack of productive assets and resources. Lack of income.	Low productivity, harvest failure, lack of markets, price fluctuations, low purchasing power and poor economic policies.
Social and human	Illness, death, old age, disability, ignorance.	Epidemics, social stigma, discrimination (gender, age, ethnicity).
	Lack of individual social capital.	Breakdown of social ties, witchcraft accusations, violence and inequality.
Natural		Drought, floods, pest attack, land degradation. Earthquakes and fires.
Political		Exclusion from civic matters, bad governance, insecurity, conflicts, riots and corruption

Source: Adapted and modified from Moser (1996).

people's vulnerability and the way they cope with and adjust to stresses. In response to socio-economic and ecological vulnerability, people living under these conditions may work together to achieve a common goal or vision (see Figure 2.1). This is a social vision that is linked to collective actions based on the social capital of a certain community. The process of developing a social vision requires that groups of individuals identify and raise issues publicly. The community discusses alternative solutions, considers their impacts, engages in implementation and provision of solutions, provides for sanctions, resolves conflicts, and monitors and evaluates outcomes. This interactive process of identification of alternatives, discussion, contestation and decision-making builds social capital (Rudd, 2000). Social vision development is a direct democratic process that leads to concrete human actions where persons take responsibility for their own action and their role in collective decisions. Communities have capabilities to interact and organize themselves to generate benefits for its members. In line with Brons *et al.* (2007), I posit that there is a need to address coping responses at the collective level, and this study attempts to assess how the community as a collective copes with HIV/AIDS impacts and increasing vulnerability in the study area.

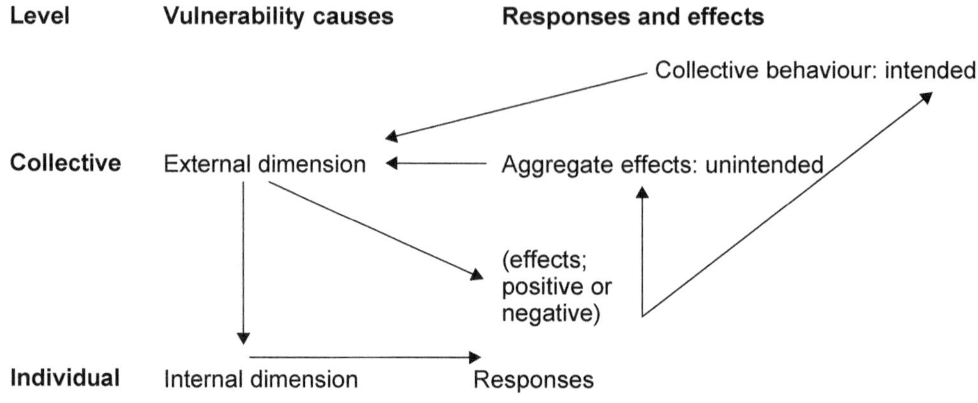

Figure 2.1. Dimensions of vulnerability (Brons et al.*, 2007).*

2.2.4. Coping strategies

The concept of coping strategy has become an important tool in food and livelihood security analysis. Although the importance of coping strategies have been long recognized, they figured prominently in the study of the aftermath of the famines in the Sahel and the Horn Africa in the mid-1980s as a means of understanding why some people survived periods of dearth while others did not. Famines also raised important debates on the issue of entitlement: the right to access resources (Sen, 1981), which is an important determinant for coping with contingencies. Many studies use the concept of coping to analyze household responses to a variety of adversities, such as those associated with natural disasters, changes in the labour market, wars, or changes at individual level such as illness or death. Davies (1993) makes the distinction between coping strategies (short-term response to an immediate food insufficiency) and adaptive strategies (long-term or permanent changes in the way in which households and individuals acquire sufficient food or income). Coping strategies are also used by individuals or communities to respond to changing environmental and socio-economic conditions or as responses to their consequences, such as declining food availability and changes in household composition. Davies (1993) notes a number of drawbacks to the use of coping strategies in food security research. Generally is a 'catch-all' term used to describe everything that rural households do apart from their primary productive activities. In most cases coping strategies are associated with success rather than with failure of livelihood systems, so are positively biased. Coping is defined as the ability to deal successfully with the stress, success implying that individuals or households are able to escape from insecurity and keep their livelihoods sustainable.

The term strategy is defined by Crowe (1989:19) as 'the presence of conscious and rational decision involving a long-term perspective'. Strategies are bound up with decisions about the use and distribution of resources. In this case, it is assumed that an individual makes a choice between two or more alternatives after performing a utility analysis. Anderson *et al.* (1994:20) define strategy as the 'overall way in which individuals, and possibly collectively, consciously seek to structure, in a coherent way, action within a relatively long-term perspective'. A combined use of both concepts - coping and strategies may be misleading to what is actually happening when individuals or households are dealing with crises. When households are responding to crises, they rarely take the long-term perspective into account (McCrone, 1994). Anderson *et al.* (1994) and McCrone (1994) in their study on household economies in Scotland noted that only better-off families perceived themselves as having better control over resources and being able to make choices and plan while the others did not. Moreover, people behaved more or less strategically at different points in the life course, meaning that they do plan at a certain stage and at another stage they do not.

Rugalema (2000) and Davies (1993) argue that using the term coping strategies tends to obscure the real experience and suffering of individuals, households and communities. The term has limited capacity to explain failure to cope. In the advent of HIV/AIDS most households do not act according to predetermined plans but rather respond to the immediate needs, in many cases incurring short and long-term costs that compromise future livelihood security. I concur with Gillespie & Loevinsohn (2003) that the term response is more appropriate than coping strategy as it brings out all the viable and non-viable, conscious and unconscious actions the households apply to manage contingencies. Therefore, the concept of coping strategy should be used with caution. Not all coping responses individuals or households employ are successful, neither do they all involve strategic decisions. In fact, coping could be an indication that things are getting worse. For instance, in responding to food insecurity, a household may apply measures that lead to nutritional deficiency of its members. In the case of HIV/AIDS impacts, dissolution of the household is an indicator of failure to cope. Barnett & Whiteside (2002) argue that people who are forced to sell the clothes of the dead or their own clothes can hardly be said to be coping - these are desperate actions.

A key aspect in handling a crisis is household assets management. Individuals, households and communities may change their mix of productive activities, and modify their community rules and institutions over the long term in response to economic, social or environmental shocks or stresses in order to meet livelihood needs. At the household level, asset base and life-course factors that affect the structure and composition of the household such as birth, marriage and death, can affect the ability to respond. Livelihood processes are highly gendered, as are the activities of women and men in responding or coping. Gender roles and relations structure responses to specific shocks and stresses. Household asymmetries in rights and obligations on the basis of gender and age translate into differential ability to cope with economic difficulties (Sen, 1990; Moser, 1993). Women, for example, may be constrained by social and cultural structures that place them in inferior social positions, limiting their access to income, education, public voice, and coping. Due to socially and culturally grounded roles, men and women have different options and responsibilities in livelihood generation as well as in the way they deal with uncertainties and risks (Niehof, 2004a).

The way households shuffle their assets and come up with responses are determined by their internal and external relations. Women play a key role in the maintenance and reproduction of the household for which they devise coping strategies which sometimes will work out at their own expense. A study conducted by IFAD (1998) in Nepal identified several of women's responses as being at their disadvantage and having a negative impact on their health. These responses included reducing their own food intake and that of their daughters, sharing food surplus between households, purchasing cheaper staples to replace costlier and more nutritious items, and working harder and longer to earn cash for buying food. When it comes to the use of extra-household relations as a coping response, reliance on informal networks is necessary among women and their households to share resources, stabilize incomes, and reduce risks. This is especially important because women tend to be poorly represented in the formal sectors and often lack access to the information that might help them survive and/or thrive. As a consequence, women have become accustomed to relying on informal networks. In the advent of HIV/AIDS the role of women's informal social networks becomes stronger, as documented for Uganda by Barnett & Blaikie (1992). In Tanzania, associations mostly operated by women involve activities like visiting orphans, widows and the sick and holding meetings at which members make contributions in cash or food. Some villagers provide labour to assist in the repair of dwellings and the rehabilitation of farms or equipment (Lwihula, 1999). Most analyses of women's capacity to cope tend to simply differentiate between men and women, often implying that they operate in separate livelihood spheres (Davies, 1996). Greater attention needs to be paid to women's ability to cope and the diversity of intra-household relations which determines causes and patterns of vulnerability.

Coping strategies and responses vary according to vulnerability status and are influenced by asset ownership. Poor households are more vulnerable than well-off ones. In developing countries coping strategies and responses of the poor are often already strained because of a number of problems including HIV/AIDS, increasing population pressure, and detrimental forces of globalization. Coping strategies are not necessarily viable or sustainable (see above). De Waal (1989) distinguishes between erosive and non-erosive coping in order to differentiate those strategies which erode the subsistence base of the household and those which do not. Some of the coping strategies used by the household may reduce flexibility and make them more vulnerable when the next crisis comes (Ellis, 2000). In the face of HIV/AIDS, some households pursue a combination of coping strategies that jeopardize the household's resilience to future shocks, thereby increasing the possibility of spiraling into increased poverty (SADC/FANR, 2003). Examples are distress sales of assets, commercial sex, withdrawing children from school and reducing food intake.

Mingione (1987) draws a distinction between coping strategies that focus on making better use of internal household resources and those that focus on mobilizing external resources provided by the state, the local community, relatives, friends, or by private organizations such as the church and ethnic groups. For both types of strategies, a difference can then be made between monetary and non-monetary resources. Monetary resources include earnings from formal or informal institutions and even individuals. Non-monetary resources include activities by household members to meet their needs through social relations of mutual support, which are the main focus of this study and are labeled social capital. Social relations feature prominently in collective social security arrangements and safety nets.

2.2.5 Collective arrangements and safety nets

Exposure to risks is a major threat in the day-to-day life of the people in developing countries. Illness, disability, death, widowhood and natural disasters are some examples of typical risks, which lead to fluctuating incomes, thereby affecting livelihoods and quality of life. Since livelihood security encompasses freedom from all dimensions of poverty and vulnerability, social security is an important concern. Social security arrangements are collective arrangements that mobilize resources for the protection and safeguarding of individual livelihoods (Midgley, 1995). A social security arrangement, however, should be based on an understanding of the strategies of individuals and households and their way of accessing resources (Nooteboom, 2003). Whereas in developed countries more than 90 percent of the populations are by now covered by various forms of state or market-organized social security systems, in developing countries a large percentage of the population remains uncovered against basic risks (Jutting, 1999). Therefore, the only alternative is to develop and utilize informal social security arrangements. As Braun (1991) remarks: for social security provision developing countries are poor in state institutions but may be rich in community institutions. However, these may not always be effective. An individual's basic support network consists of relations with kin and family as well as with neighbours and friends that provide entitlements defined through mutual responsibility and reciprocity. Such networks have always been important for differential access to various means of existence (Baerends, 1994; Agarwal, 1991). Social claims are extra-household resource, which offer a source of security to individuals and households particularly in times of need.

In this study, I define social security as the collective arrangements of a group to protect the livelihood of its members against the threats of shocks and stress. I will focus on locally organized forms of social security commonly referred to as informal social security. These community-based social security arrangements are based on systems of mutual dependence and reciprocity. They are social mechanisms for preventing contingencies, such as a decrease in income, sickness and crop failure, alleviating their effects, and protecting vulnerable social groups in the community. Platteau (1991:113) summarizes that:

> *'Social arrangements and economic institutions in the traditional village societies have thus been especially designed to cope with the threat of hunger and other kinds of contingencies. The fact of the matter is that the moral economy of traditional rural communities can be largely interpreted as social security economy, in that people belonging to these communities are able to find collective methods to protect themselves against major contingencies and production hazards.'*

These social arrangements need not to take the form of a special program, but are embedded in the economic organization and social relations. However, it should be noted that informal social security arrangements do not always provide equal access for all members in the community, which shows that they do not always succeed in providing the overall security as intended. Collective social arrangements are about risk management. People living in an ecologically uniform area, carrying out more or less similar activities, face the same risks and have little to gain by sharing or pooling their risks. This is called covariate risk. A study conducted on the changing patterns of resource use in local agrarian systems in Kenya, Ghana, Nigeria and Zambia during and after the colonial period illustrates the limits of informal social security arrangements. 'Impoverishment and instability often affect whole families and communities, undermining their ability to provide security for any, let alone all of their members', says Berry (1993:195). This is very much applicable to Tanzania where sharing risks and coping through mutual insurance is strained because of various forces.

The clustered nature of HIV/AIDS adds to the epidemic's feature as a covariate risk, where reliance on social networks to mitigate its impacts becomes less of an option. HIV/AIDS does not affect persons at random in the household or community: the

infection and impacts are clustered. The clustering of HIV/AIDS within the household is a consequence of both sexual relations and mother-to-child transmission. It exerts a cumulative impact, affecting the composition of the household in a way that is not easy to repair (Baylies, 2002). Families live with HIV, not just individuals (Rotheram-Borus *et al.*, 2005). If an individual in the household is affected, the impacts of the epidemic are shared through kinship relations, neighbourhood relations and other social relations within and between households. As the epidemic unfolds, household and family structures are affected and these changes are extended to the community, exerting an increasing strain.

Examples of collective social security arrangements include burial societies, grain-saving schemes, labour-sharing clubs, and rotating saving-and-credit associations. Different studies show the importance of such arrangements and describe the extent to which those in need turn to these groups for assistance (Rugalema, 1999; Madembo 1997; Topouzis & Hemrich, 1996). In Kagera, Tanzania, Lundberg *et al.* (2000) found that assistance to households following the death of an adult came from private transfers offered by relatives and friends. Lwihula (1999) found that in addition to the pre-existing traditional saving and mutual assistance association, in many villages, particularly in the hardest hit areas, people launched new organizations specifically aimed at coping with the costs of the AIDS epidemic, providing assistance to members in the event of death and sickness. Women typically play a significant role in the cultivation of social relationships and are instrumental in arranging complex reciprocal gift-giving systems. These support structures have proved to be important for women (Agarwal, 1991; Ardener, 1995).

Other studies have urged that there are limits to such assistance, and that kinship networks and extended family structures of reciprocity must be realistically seen as safety nets with holes. Not all individuals and households are supported, whether because of their weak kinship ties or as a consequence of the stigma represented by AIDS. The strength of social support networks also varies with the overall resource base of those involved in the interactions. Poor networks will have little to offer to their members and in any case entitlements vary according to one's position in the network, with some being able to claim more than others (Baylies, 2002). It was found that in Kagera, Tanzania, poor households have very little to offer when tragedy occurs (Lundberg *et al.,* 2000). The ability of the poorest people to maintain wider reciprocal relations beyond their immediate household is constrained because of their lack of means (Cleaver, 2005). Although it has been documented that many of the households affected by HIV/AIDS receive assistance from friends and neighbours, Rakodi (1999) and Sauerborn *et al.* (1996) noted that as assets at household level become depleted, there is much less contribution to mutual and collective arrangements within the community.

2.3 Social capital

The role of social capital at micro and macro levels in the process of economic development and poverty reduction is increasingly emphasized in the literature, acknowledging that lack of or changes in social capital may hinder social and economic development (Dhesi, 2000). Previous studies have commented on its economic and social significance, such as the relationship between the distribution of social capital and household incomes (Narayan & Pritchett, 1999) and social capital as safety nets (Morduch, 1999). Studies show that the quantity, quality and persistence of social interactions among neighbours, friends and members of groups and associations, generate social capital and the ability to work together for a common good, which is especially important for the poor (Grootaert *et al.*, 1999; Morduch 1999; Moser, 1998). Wider social relationships and the degree of social cohesion in the community may affect individual's health and feelings of safety (Wilkinson, 2002). Knack & Keefer (1997) examined market economies and found that investments and growth rates were higher in countries where interpersonal trust and norms of civic cooperation were greater. They also found that trust and cooperation are well developed in countries with well-developed legal institutions to protect property and contract rights and in countries that are relatively homogeneous in terms of income and social levels.

Social capital is regarded as particularly important as a last resort resource for the poor and vulnerable. It can provide a buffer that helps them cope with shocks, such as death in the family, functioning as an informal safety net to ensure survival during periods of intense insecurity and compensating for a lack of other types of capital (e.g. labour groups compensating for limited human capital within the household). Social capital provided by family and close friends provides assistance and care and also creates a sense of well-being. In HIV/AIDS situation, social capital has been said to facilitate households to respond its impacts. As social capital is the main focus of this study it is discussed in more detail than other household assets.

People constantly interact with other people who might provide access to resources and support at times of need. When it comes to support and survival, personal relationships and social networks are crucial. The capabilities to mobilize social relations and networks of personal benefits and support are captured in the term social capital. Much interest in the concept perhaps stems from its perceived positive consequences for development, its character as a non-monetary source of power, influence and information, and from the opportunities it provides for those who lack possession of and access to other forms of capital such as financial, human or natural. As Portes (1998) observes, whereas economic capital is in people's bank accounts and human capital is inside their heads, social capital inheres in the structure of their relationships. Social capital is created from the myriad of everyday interactions between people. Drawing on the work of Bourdieu (1985) and Coleman (1988), Portes (1998) argues that social capital resides in the relationships between actors. As a relational concept, social capital exists only as far as several individuals share it. Where people share a sense of identity, hold similar values, trust each other and reciprocally do things for each other, there will be a positive impact on the social, political and economic organization of the community they are living in. Thus, social relationships can lead to the development of norms of trust and reciprocity that have a spill-over effect within the community as whole. The role of social capital has evolved into it being a panacea for the problems that affect societies (Portes, 1998), although this is evidently not the case (Fine, 2001; Portes & Landolt, 1996; Putzel, 1997).

The concept of social capital had been greatly stimulated by the writings of James Coleman (1988; 1990) and Robert Putnam (1993). The broad definition of social capital distinguishes two forms of social capital to cover its structural and cognitive aspects. Structurally, social capital implies networks or social structures in which people are embedded. These are structures that are observable. Cognitive social capital refers to contents such as trust, shared beliefs, norms of obligation and reciprocity. These are intangible and subjective (Uphoff & Wijayaratna, 2000). Putnam (1993) defined social capital in terms of horizontal social groups such as associations, clubs and voluntary agencies that bring individuals together to pursue one or more objectives in which they have a common interest, e.g. farmers associations. Coleman (1990:598) defines social capital as 'a variety of different entities (which) all consist of some aspects of social structure, and (which) facilitate certain actions of actors - whether personal or corporate actors - within the structure'. In this definition he considered relations among groups rather than individuals and includes vertical components. North (1990) cited in Berger-Schmitt (2000) introduced an even more comprehensive perspective of social capital, which includes formalized relations and structures of macro-institutions, such as the political regime or the legal and judicial systems. Corresponding to these different dimensions of the concept, a distinction between three levels of manifestation can be made:

- Interpersonal relations, such as family, friends and neighbours.
- Intermediary associations and organizations such as clubs, forms, political parties.
- Macro-level societal institutions, extending to formal institutions and relationships and structures, such as government, the political regime, the rule of law, the court system, and civil and political autonomy. This is the social and political environment that shapes social structure and enables norms and trust to develop.

There is a very strong degree of complementary and substitution between these three levels and their coexistence maximizes the impact of social capital on economic and social outcomes (Grootaert & Bastelaer, 2002).

A key element of social capital is the notion of more or less densely interlocking networks of relationships between individuals and groups. Networks can be more or less formal. There is a widespread consensus in the literature that formal and informal networks coexist and supplement each other (Groat, 1997). Stone & Hughes (2001) argue that informal networks based on personal ties can emerge from involvement in formal networks because they foster repeated interaction among people with common interests. To distinguish between the two, legal recognition and organizational structure are used. Informal social networks comprise face-to-face relationships between a limited number of individuals who know each other and are bound together by kinship, friendship or another type of close relationship. In most cases, the members of these networks have some form of mutual interests. However, membership in these networks is rather fluid. It should be noted that these networks often are institutionalized through deeply embedded patterns of social practices and norms (Weissmann, 2005). They lack legal recognition, full-time officials, written rules, and hierarchy. Thus, the characteristic outputs of informal networks consists of small-scale do-it-yourself services, such as helping in repairing the house, child care, helping in cultivation, moral support at time of difficulties, etc. (Rose, 1999). Most outputs are based on affection or obligation within a family, extended family or friendship network.

It is their structure that distinguishes informal networks from formal ones. Formal networks tend to be more complex and hierarchically organized. A formal network is one that is set up with specific members and objectives and is officially recognized. They always have specific goals that need to be met. Formal networks tend to have more clearly demarcated boundaries than informal ones. They have rules and procedures for entrance, membership, and expulsion. Formal networks have a set of rules and a number of officers who operate in their name and roles are usually predetermined and assigned to members. Each role will have specific responsibilities and duties. The advantage of informal networks over formal networks is that they are highly adaptive and responsive to best deal with urgent local problems; they may be more easily changed to meet specific circumstances. For the purpose of this study formal networks are defined as social networks of individuals in which the individuals involved explicitly agree on the objectives, rules, procedures, and activities. Informal networks are defined as social connections of individuals without formal structures, linked together by kinship, friendship, ethnicity or neighbourhood.

Both formal and informal networks are embedded in the prevailing power structures within a given community. Since women are less likely to participate in the formal wage sector and to belong to formal organizations, they are more likely to rely on kin and social networks for access to resources. Hence, informal networks and social relationships are particularly important for women. Social networks often operate along gender lines, although the literature tends to treat them as gender-neutral institutions (Dikito-Wachtmeister, 2001; Molyneux, 2002). The research of Silvey & Elmhirst (2003) on women workers and rural-urban networks in Indonesia revealed that while social networks provide distinct advantages, at the same time they demand particular contributions from women in different contexts. In most cases women and men belong to different social networks, whereby women's networks cannot command and exercise as much authority as those of men. In such situations, social networks may further isolate women from mainstream decision-making and this may affect their livelihood-generation.

The benefits and costs of participation in social networks are unequally distributed. One does not acquire or squander social capital on the basis of individual choice, one rather accrues obligation and opportunity to participate in social networks by virtue of one's position (Rankin, 2002). This has great implications for women's ability to benefit from and participate in the networks. Because of socio-economic and cultural reasons, women may be deprived from participating in and benefiting from social networks. Some studies show that females have considerable a social capital deficit as compared to their male counterparts (Mayoux, 2001; Molyneux, 2002). To build social capital women depend on time and resources of which they tend to have less than men. Gender inequality has negative effects on the use and generation of social capital. Gender inequality limits trust, hinders family relations, restricts social networks, and depletes social assets, which are the valuable resource of societies to work toward common goals (Picciotto, 1998). Since social networks exist within a broader context of gender inequality, this study assesses gender aspects by looking at the ways which women and men access food and cope with impacts of HIV/AIDS through social networks.

Social capital does not imply the immediate and formally accounted exchange of the legal or business contract, but is a combination of short-term altruism and long-term self-interest (Lyon, 2000). Individuals provide a service to others or act for the benefit of others, doing this in the general expectation that it will be returned at some undefined time in the future when they might need it themselves. Trust entails a willingness to take risks in a social context, in the confidence that others will respond as expected and will act in mutually supportive ways. Fukuyama (1995:26) defined trust as the expectation within a community of regular, honest and cooperative behaviour, based on commonly shared norms on the part of other members of that community. Social norms provide a form of informal social control that remove the need for more formal, institutionalized legal sanctions. Social norms are unwritten but commonly understood. They determine what patterns of behaviour are expected in a given social context, and define what forms of behaviour is socially approved and how specific behaviour is valued.

Putman (2000) distinguishes two types of social relationships: bonding and bridging. He describes the first as a relationship between similar or homogenous people, such as the relations among families. Bonding connectedness occurs within one's core community, and therefore reinforces exclusive identities along gender lines, class, etc. Bonding social capital enables individuals or households to fulfill their daily needs and overcome difficulties. Bridging refers to those relationships between people of unequal economic status or social class, from a different generation or different social groups. Bridging relationships are extended beyond one's immediate environment, hence broadening social connectedness and experiences across diverse social associations. The ties in bridging social networks tend to be weaker and diverse, but are more important for 'getting ahead'. Woolcock (2000) identified a third type of social relationship, linking social capital, which refers to connections with people in positions of power and is characterized by relations between those within a hierarchy but at differing levels of power. The capacity to gain access to resources, ideas and information from formal institutions beyond the community is a key function of linking social capital. A relationship with a patron or chief is also considered to be linking social capital, because of the claims that can be made at time of crisis. It is different from bonding and bridging in that it is concerned with vertical relations where people involved are not equal.

Although there is consensus over social capital as being social and collective, there is still debate on the question of whether social capital is a form of capital. Social capital shares some fundamental attributes with other forms of capital, while there are also some that differ. Like other capital, social capital is productive, yielding outcomes such as information sharing and collective action. Like physical capital, social capital requires regular maintenance, in the form of repeated social interaction or trust building behaviour (Grootaert & Bastelaer, 2002). Ostrom (1999) noted that investment in physical capital is usually based on a conscious decision, while social capital may be developed as a by-product of other activities as well as being purposeful. Arrow (1999) has objected to the use of capital on the grounds that it suggests a misleading analogy with physical capital. Investment in physical capital always involves foregoing current benefits for future gains, and physical capital can be sold or otherwise transferred to others. Neither is necessarily true of social capital. Unlike physical capital (but like human capital) social capital is depleted with its disuse. Social capital being social cannot be built-up individually, unlike human capital. In spite of disagreement on the use of term 'capital' among different disciplines, Grootaert & Bastelacr (2002) observed that it offers a unique opportunity for cooperation in multidisciplinary research and development activities.

The use of social capital tends to be identified with only positive outcomes, which is increasingly questioned as being too normative (Adler & Kwon, 1999). Investments in social capital, like investments in physical capital, are not costless, and therefore unbalanced investment or over-investment in social capital can transform a potentially productive asset into a constraint and a liability. The enthusiasm about the 'bright side' of social capital, neglects the fact that social networks may at times have detrimental effects on the actors involved. Instead of helping they may hinder their ability to pursue their interests (Portes & Sensenbrenner, 1993). Social capital can turn sour (Moerbeek, 2001). Other identified negative consequences of social capital include exclusion of outsiders, excess claims on the group members, restriction on individual freedom, and a downward leveling norm (Portes, 1998; Adler & Kwon, 1999).

Because social capital is a multifaceted concept, measuring it and its effects is difficult. Empirical studies have used a wide range of variables as indicators of social capital. Conceptual vagueness, the coexistence of multiple definitions, and the chronic lack of suitable data have been impediments to both theoretical and empirical research on the subject (Sabatini, 2005). Social capital measurement is also considerably complicated by the fact that social capital research has frequently relied upon measures of the outcomes of social capital as indicators of social capital itself (Stone, 2001). Moreover, most studies measure social capital only quantitatively not qualitatively, but both the quantity and quality are relevant to its usefulness (UKONS, 2001). Some studies use one indicator of social capital, such as civic associations, that fails to adequately capture the multifaceted nature of the concept (Stone, 2001). Most empirical research on social capital has been concerned with formal networks, mainly because they are easy to identify. Grootaert & Bastelaer (2002) suggest developing methodologies that will cover the four quadrants shown in Figure 2.2 when studying social capital.

In summary, social capital focuses on networks: the relationships within and between them, and the norms which govern these relationships. As with poverty, entitlement and the livelihood approach, the concept of social capital has been applied in many contexts, and refers to social problems and vulnerability of people. In poverty studies, it is commonly argued that while poor people lack material assets, they can generally call on close relations with family, neighbours and friends as a form of social security. Woolcock (2000) argues that poor people typically have plenty of bonding social capital. In the literature, social capital is largely seen as comprising claims, rights and possibilities that people have and does not represent a fixed and

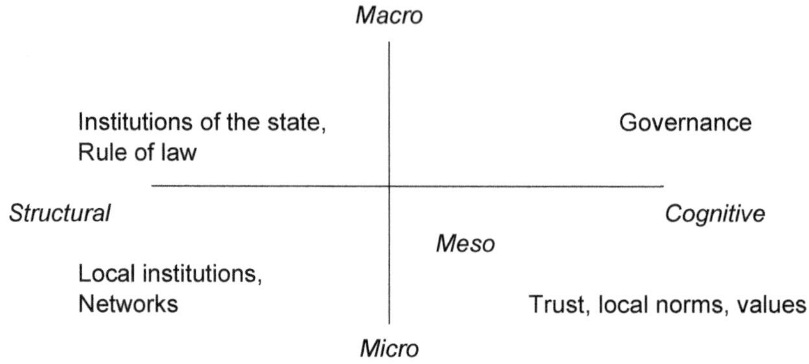

Figure 2.2. Forms and scope of social capital (Grootaert & Bastelaer, 2002).

certain body of capital that can be cashed in at times of need. It does not give an indication of how these possibilities are harnessed or mobilized. It does not even explain why some people are less vulnerable than others and why some people receive more support than others. There has been a neglect of hierarchy in social capital research by not addressing power issues. Furthermore, the linkages between the micro- and meso-level are not well explored and demonstrated.

In the context of this study, the concept of social capital is used to describe activities in everyday life which involve participation in social networks to meet individual and household needs and the associated norms and values that underlie these networks. The study applies the concept both in terms of its structural aspects (social relations and networks) and its cognitive dimension (shared values and trust). Social capital can be both directly and indirectly beneficial to the households. First, it is a resource facilitating access to other resources. Secondly, it is an asset in terms of claims to immediate support, whether material or non-material. Despite its drawbacks, social capital may enable households affected by HIV/AIDS to cope with and mitigate its impacts. I argue that investment in social networks enhances the rights of an individual or household to draw or claim on them when needed. Therefore, critical assessment should be made on how social capital functions in the context of HIV/AIDS.

As the focus of this study is on the micro-level of the household, the emphasis is on individuals' and households' abilities to mobilize resources through social networks like kinship networks, friends, neighbours and community groups. The study analyzes how individuals and households are coping with HIV/AIDS impacts and other contingencies by relying on interpersonal relationships and community groups. Social capital at micro-level interfaces with social capital at meso-level which is why community-level social interaction and organization and community-level trust are investigated. It is recognized that access to social capital is influenced by the wider socio-cultural and economic context in which social networks function. The social context plays an important role in the generation of social capital. In livelihood studies contextual factors are associated with the external dimension of vulnerability and those at individual level are related to the internal dimension. The two dimensions are linked to each other and affect responses at both individual and community levels, as shown in Figure 2.1.

Community and civil society

Peoples' social interactions enable them to build communities, to commit themselves to each other, and to knit the social fabric (Beem, 1999). The nature of the relationships between people and the social networks which they are a part of is often seen as one of the more significant aspects of community. Trust and reciprocity among community members determine the quality of community life (Putnam, 1993, 2000). As Hawton *et al.* (1999) noted communities are not homogenous entities; they are differentiated through ethnicity, gender and class, and may contain diverse groups whose interests may conflict with each other.

There are different ways to define community: as a group of people living in a particular place or as an area of common life. In most cases there is overlap in that people who live in a particular location share common interests and visions. Cohen (1985) argues that communities are best approached as 'communities of meaning', to be identified by their symbolic boundaries. The association that a particular group of people have with each other and with the space they occupy is embedded in people's lives and is enacted through activities such as work and religious rituals (Bourque, 1997). A community becomes distinct in relation to another community. Cohen (1985) argues that community involves two related suggestions namely that the members of a group have something in common with each other, and that what they have in common distinguishes them in a significant way from the members of other groups. Cohen (1985:15) notes that even though people share symbols, they do not necessarily share the same meanings. Symbolic boundaries are perceived in different ways by people on either side of the boundary (Cohen, 1985:12). People create their own communities within the context of a specific cultural and political environment. This may mean that multiple communities may exist within one place. Special social and cultural characteristics of life, for example language, ethnic identity, rituals, social class or a combination of these, may symbolically define a community. Other characteristics of community may be based upon gender, religion, or a mutually shared issue or problem. These characteristics may also include a sense of inclusiveness and belonging. Conversely, it may also mean exclusion to others.

Communities are important because at community-level issues and problems can be addressed that cannot be handled either by individuals acting alone or by markets and governments. It is social capital that enables community members to work for the common good. In communities with a high level of social capital, people are able to provide something of value to other members of the community. Community connectedness makes a big difference in many aspects of human life. Putnam (2000) notes that social capital makes us smarter, healthier, safer, richer and better able to govern a just and stable democracy. Strong communities that are characterized by social equality, mutual caring and support, and social cohesion, reduce a population's vulnerability to AIDS (Decosas, 2002).

Communities in the social sense are part of civil society. Although there is no universally accepted definition of civil society, it generally thought to refer to the sphere of voluntary social association, which is outside both the state and the family (Harris, 2001; Perlas, 2000). A conceptualization of civil society that is well applicable to the African context is provided by Orvis (2001:19). He defines civil society as 'a public sphere of formal or informal collective activity, autonomous from but recognizing the legitimate existence of the state and family'. This definition allows the inclusion of traditional or ethnic organizations, self-help and cooperative groups, patronage networks, and traditional authorities as viable elements of civil society. The role of the civil society in relationship to the state can differ. In some cases they can be seen as a countervailing power, in other cases or as mutually interdependent in relation to the state, and their relationship to the state as antagonistic or complementary (Beauclerk & Heap, 2003). Jamil & Muriisa (2004) contend that civil society works well in a peaceful political environment and perhaps with a synergic relation with the state rather than with the state interfering in its activities.

Sometimes civil society is equated with social capital, but these two concepts are not the same. Civil society represents non-governmental institutional arrangements, while social capital describes the social relationships from which these institutional arrangements emerge. Civil society forms the context within which social capital is nurtured. Therefore, social capital is an integral part of civil society. As people interact in a community they establish norms, learn to trust each other and commit themselves to providing help for each other, thus establishing civic consciousness needed for political participation and economic development (Putnam, 2000). Trust and willingness to cooperate allows people to form groups and associations, which facilitate the realization of shared goals. Civil society does not include behaviour imposed or even coerced by the state. Civil society commonly embraces a diversity of spaces, actors and institutional forms, varying in their degree of formality, autonomy and power. Civil society is made up of organizations such as NGOs, self-help community groups, religious organizations, professional associations, trades unions and advocacy groups.

Meso-level social capital is a key component of the study. To be able to investigate the role of meso-level social capital and its interface with micro-level social capital in the mitigation of AIDS-impacts, it has to be put in a concrete context. Within the scope of this study meso-level social capital was anchored at a community in the geographic and social sense. The administrative unit of the village, which is a geographic cluster of a number of hamlets, was used to investigate the significance of community-level social capital and civil society for individuals' and households' coping with the impacts of HIV/AIDS.

2.4 Conceptual framework of the study

Based on the preceding theoretical discussion, a model (Figure 2.3) was developed to show HIV/AIDS impacts, household livelihood and social capital interaction.

This model guided the research and facilitated the implementation of the study. Basically there are three clusters of relationships that are involved. The first cluster (1) concerns the direct impacts of HIV/AIDS on household resources and assets. The second cluster (2) comprises the indirect impacts of HIV/AIDS, operating through social capital at both interpersonal and community level. The third cluster (3) involves implications of AIDS impacts for household livelihood, under which food security and care are subsumed. The household is placed at the centre of the

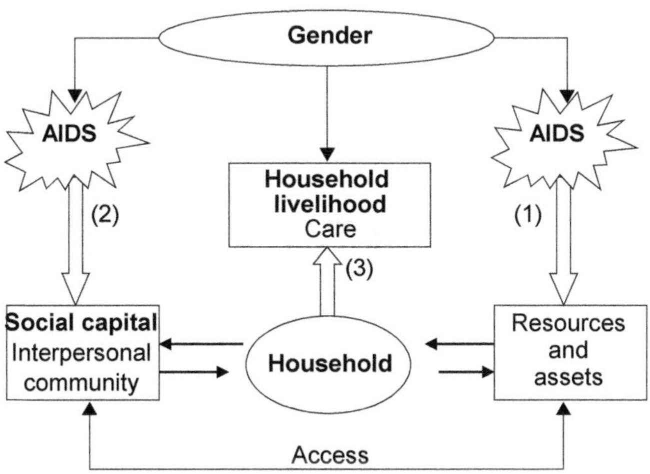

Figure 2.3. The relationship between HIV/AIDS, social capital and household livelihood.

model, because it is the locus where resource management for livelihood takes place and where HIV/AIDS impacts are pointedly felt. Gender is given a central position because we know from the literature that these processes are gendered.

Chapter 3
Research design and methodology

This chapter gives a detailed account on how the study was conducted. It describes the rationale behind the research design, the unit of analysis, and the sampling procedures and methods used in data collection. Important methodological issues of validity and reliability and ethical considerations are discussed as well.

3.1 Study site

As explained in Chapter 2, the need to investigate meso-level social capital and its interface with micro-level social capital in mitigating HIV/AIDS impacts in a given context necessitated the choice of one village. To be able to investigate in great detail the process and mechanisms through which AIDS mortality and morbidity changes social capital that individuals have or might generate to ensure sustainable livelihood it was necessary to focus on just one village. To be able to capture changes and observe evolving events, it was important to have a long stay in the village. Because the study involved sensitive topics like HIV/AIDS and food security it was important for the researcher to interact regularly and intensively with community members so as to gain their confidence. Therefore, focusing the research on one village was the logical and necessary choice.

The research was conducted in a village called Mkamba in Kilombero District, Tanzania. In Tanzania, a village is the second lowest government administrative unit. It consists of several hamlets, with the hamlet being the smallest administrative unit. The term village is used to refer to rural localities only. Mkamba village was purposively selected on the basis of a reconnaissance visit to the area in January 2004. The criteria used for selecting the research area were:

- Relatively high HIV/AIDS prevalence rates with a potential to capture the impacts of HIV/AIDS for various households. Information obtained from Morogoro Regional Hospital officials and available HIV/AIDS data at regional level, showed Kilombero District to have relatively high HIV/AIDS prevalence. Further discussions with medical and other district officials led to the choice of Mkamba.
- Varied livelihood portfolios. Based on the information of district officials it could be ascertained that in Mkamba village though livelihoods are based on agriculture people engage in a variety of livelihood activities.

However, the research area was not confined to this village only as other villages were considered when issues of exchange and family relations were investigated. During the research two other issues transpired. The first issue was that privatization of the sugarcane plantation (in 1998) had seriously affected people's access to agricultural land and income. This will be further explained in Chapter 4. The second was that with respect to village organization and the strength of civil society a neighbouring village (Kidatu) proved to provide a much more positive picture than Mkamba. Therefore, it was deemed necessary to collect information on Kidatu, to be able to assess the extent to which Mkamba village presents a special case and in what respects it might be a special case. Hence, key informants from Kidatu village were interviewed about its general characteristics, including access to land, and the social organization and community initiatives in the village.

3.2 Research design

The nature of the problem under study necessitated applying a longitudinal perspective and using a combination of qualitative and quantitative methods, to be able to uncover household processes in livelihood generation and social capital formation in the wake of the HIV/AIDS epidemic.

3.2.1 Longitudinal approach

A longitudinal approach adds the dimension of time to the analysis of the household's different patterns of responses to various events in its life course (Pennartz & Niehof, 1999). The nature of HIV/AIDS as a long wave shock (Barnett & Blaikie, 1992; Booysen & Arntz, 2003) calls for a longitudinal perspective. Its slow incubation period, its demographic and down-spiraling socio-economic consequences, which are likely to last for more than one generation, also calls for a longitudinal perspective. Secondly, household composition as an important determinant of social-economic achievement changes over time. A life-course perspective is relevant in studying the household, because household labour availability and productivity are strongly related to the stages in the household life-course. It is difficult to capture a full range of effects and coping responses within a cross-sectional study. However, due to financial and time constraints this study could only incorporate a longitudinal perspective by following up on already existing information or data on the research area, and by asking retrospective questions and documenting life histories. Repeated observation on same cases enabled the researcher to observe short-term changes occurring in the households.

3.2.2 Combining qualitative and quantitative methods

The nature of the study necessitated a combination of qualitative and quantitative methods of data collection and analysis so as to gain deeper understanding of the phenomena under study. Qualitative and quantitative methods complement each other, and their combined application optimizes both reliability and validity (Scrimshaw, 1990; Niehof, 1999). The integration of qualitative and quantitative methods allowed the researcher to understand the context and uncover the links between social capital and other socio-economic processes in the study area. In this study quantitative method was used to describe socio-economic, demographic and social networks information of the respondents. Qualitative methods were utilized to obtain information on actual behaviour, to interpret the meanings behind it, and to gain insight into how people experience their situation. The study employed a sequential integration of qualitative and quantitative methods. Qualitative methods such as open-ended interviews with key informants and focus group discussions (FGD) also helped in operationalizing the theoretical concepts for designing the questionnaire. At a later stage, survey findings were clarified and validated by using qualitative methods such as case study and FGD. Additionally, to investigate sensitive topics such as HIV/AIDS, gender relations and food insecurity, the use of qualitative methods brings out information that people will not disclose in a survey. In the final analysis quantitative and qualitative findings are linked and where discrepancies were noted, reasons are given.

3.3 Research units

In this study the basic research unit is the household because it is the locus of livelihood generation and it provides the daily context for coping with HIV/AIDS impacts and care (see Chapter 2).Because of intra-household differences, especially in the case studies specific individuals were subjected to in-depth interviews. For measuring meso-level social capital the community as a whole became the research unit. In between the household and the community level the interactions between households, beyond-household relationships and the context in which these relations operate were examined.

3.4 Definition of HIV/AIDS cases

Because the majority of the people are reluctant to go for a HIV test and, if they do so, they are reluctant to disclose their status, the objective assessment of people's HIV-status is problematic. However, the villagers have some indicators they use to come to the conclusion that somebody has AIDS or guess that somebody might be infected. These indicators emerged during the focus group discussions and were later used to identify some of the HIV/AIDS affected respondents. HIV/AIDS-affected individuals or households were identified as follows:

i. Assessment on the basis of death or sickness caused by common opportunistic diseases associated with HIV/AIDS, such as TB, pneumonia, frequent fevers, persistent skin problems, and chronic diarrhea.
ii. Key informants reporting of known HIV/AIDS cases and deaths in the community, of which the households were treated as HIV/AIDS affected although there was no medical evidence for this.

A household was considered HIV/AIDS-affected if it had person/s suffering from prolonged AIDS-related illnesses, it experienced members' death due to AIDS-related illnesses, or if it had AIDS-orphans in its care. By using the two approaches above, 30 households were identified as HIV/AIDS-affected out of the 180 households in the survey. Most individuals and households identified as HIV/AIDS-affected did not admit so. Out of 30 identified HIV/AIDS-affected cases, only six households disclosed AIDS as the cause of death of their household members, and in only one household people admitted to having a household member suffering from AIDS. This approach may have lead to misclassification of affected households as unaffected and on the other hand unaffected households may have, without our knowledge, included households with HIV/AIDS.

3.5 Data collection methods

So as to answer the study research questions a combination of both primary and secondary data collection methods were employed. The following section provides information about the data collection methods, their main purpose and the type of information obtained from individuals, households, institutions and secondary records (see Table 3.1).

3.5.1 Methods of primary data collection

A combination of qualitative and quantitative methods of data collection was used to achieve triangulation (i.e confirmation of the same information by different methods or sources) and increase the validity of the results. Qualitative methods used included semi-structured interviews with key informants, focus group discussions, participant observation, case studies and life histories. The quantitative methods used were the household survey and the inventory of community-level groups and associations. A short description of the methods used is presented in the following section.

i. Reconnaissance visit

The AWLAE Project facilitated the travel to Tanzania in December 2003 to identify a suitable fieldwork site and gather relevant preliminary information on the area.

Table 3.1. Overview of data collection levels and methods.

Level	Type of data	Methods
Individuals	(Changes in) access to resources, ownership of assets, supporting social relationships, and participation in community groups	Life history Genealogical method Observation In-depth interviewing Ego-centric network mapping
Household	(Changes in) resource base, livelihood, food security, involvement in support networks, participation in community groups and intra-household relations	Household survey FGDs
Community	(Changes in) community structures, norms and values related to support and reciprocity, community-level resources and organizations	Secondary sources Group inventory Key informant interviews FGDs

Specific objectives of the visit were to establish contacts with government agencies and NGOs working in the area and explore possibilities for cooperation during the study. The visit allowed collection of secondary data on socio-economic, political and cultural aspects of the area including demographic data, information on peoples' livelihood, the HIV/AIDS situation and various forms of formal and informal networks in the area.

ii. Preliminary visit

After the approval of the research proposal, back in Tanzania a preliminary visit to the village was paid for introduction and planning purposes. A meeting was held with district and village leaders and other representatives of villagers including formal groups. These were introductory meetings for planning the fieldwork in the village. Information was provided on the purpose and relevance of the study as well as on the planned duration of the fieldwork. During this visit it was possible to get general information about the village and identify research assistants and key informants who took part in the first stage of field activities.

iii. Key informant interviews

The advantage of key informants interviews was that the researcher could access confidential information, which otherwise would not been easy to get. The interviews were also used to get general information about the people and situation in the village, including the changes during the past five to ten years. Interviews with key-informant were informal and guided by open-ended questions. Sometimes the researcher explored relevant topics as the informant brought them up during the interview. Key informants were: government officials, informal leaders, religious leaders, leaders of community-based organizations (CBOs), elderly and influential people in the village, traditional healers, moneylenders, and local government staff in the area such as health officers, extension staff and community development workers. The interviews were conducted in Swahili. The issues explored included:

- Origin of the village, recent history and major events in the village.
- Administrative and leadership structures.
- People's livelihoods in the village.
- Household structures and housing.
- Gender relations.
- Social relations and communal activities.
- Witchcraft.
- HIV/AIDS situation in the village.
- Ways of coping with livelihood insecurities.

iv. Focus Group Discussion (FGD)

Focus group discussions are among the most widely used methods in qualitative research. The method takes advantage of the interaction between small groups of people. Participants respond to and build on what others in the group have said. Ideally, it is a synergetic approach that helps in generating insightful information and encourages the participants to give sincere answers. For this study, the FGDs involved people who represented different groups in the village. The groups were composed of seven to eight people of varied ages. Some were mixed others counted only women or only men. The composition of the focus groups and the topics discussed are summarized in Table 3.2.

Prior to the meeting the participants were given an invitation letter stating the objective of the meeting and the intended topics of discussion. Most discussions lasted for about 90 minutes, though the women FGDs and the one with the youth lasted longer. The youth selected were peer educators for HIV/AIDS. Because of their openness other sensitive issues like food security and transactional sex could also be freely discussed. With regards to all topics participants in the focus group

Table 3.2. Composition and topics of FGDs.

No.	Composition	Topic discussed
1	Mixed (men and women)	Livelihood/food security, major problems in the area, food security indicators, coping with problems
2	Women	Same as FGD 1
3	Men	Intra-household and gender aspects: division of labour, time use, decision making, access and control of resources
4	Women	Same as FGD 3
5	Mixed	Wealth-poverty categorization, and seasonal calendar
6	Men	Participation in social networks, groups and communal activities; rights, social claims and obligations of individuals; trust as well as changes in social relations
7	Women	Same as FGD 6
8	Mixed	HIV/AIDS issues: indicators and effects on household livelihoods
9	Youth (mixed)	Same as FGD 8
10	Men	Findings of the preliminary analysis
11	Women	Same as FGD 10

discussions were asked to compare the present situation with that of five to ten years ago. Free listing was used during focus group discussions to derive definitions of variables and indictors to be used for HIV/AID-affected status, social capital, food security and socio-economic status concepts. These definitions and indicators informed the formulation of questionnaire items. The discussions were conducted in Swahili. They were all tape-recorded and then transcribed. Translation from Swahili into English was done for the sake of further analysis.

v. Household survey

This method allows the collection of empirical data on specific variables from a large sample. However, there is a methodological challenge when the survey method is used to reveal HIV/AIDS impacts, because random sampling techniques may not yield sufficient households affected by HIV/AIDS to make meaningful comparisons with non-affected households.

The sampling frame was the entire village population. At first, systematic random sampling was planned, but it proved to be impossible to get a random sample from the village register because it was not complete and because part of those selected were not in the village during the survey period as they were in their distant farms. Additionally, there was the problem of getting sufficient affected households in the sample when using a random procedure (see above). Also a stratified random sampling procedure is not possible in a situation where there is no register of affected households. Therefore, a non-probability sampling procedure was adopted to select the sample for the household survey. The sample of 180 households was obtained by a combination of cluster and purposive sampling. Four hamlets were chosen from the six hamlets in the village, based on people's livelihood activities. The two hamlets that were not chosen are mainly composed of employees of the local sugar company and the hydro-electric power company. From the four hamlets, a proportional sample was drawn to get the number of respondents needed from each hamlet. Within the hamlets the method used to find respondents has been referred to as the 'walk-and-talk' method, meaning that the field assistants together with the enumerators walked in the area and approached potential respondents for their cooperation. To have sufficient HIV/AIDS-affected and women-headed households in the sample the help of the hamlet leaders was enlisted. Potential households were contacted prior to the interview to inform them about the purpose of the survey and get their consent. Household heads interviewed were identified as such by other household members. Table 3.3 provides the numbers of selected households per hamlet.

Non-probability sampling methods such as had to be used in the study have inherent selection biases, which make the findings not representative of the larger population. Still, Bowie *et al.* (1996) as quoted in Booysen & Arntz (2003) argue that the results from such studies should be considered indicative or instructive of certain aspects or impacts rather than as statistically representative, which is also applicable to this study.

Enumerators were trained before embarking on their interviews. Questionnaire pre-testing was done with a team of trained enumerators. Some adjustments were

Table 3.3. Number of households selected for the survey.

Hamlet name	Total population	Number of households chosen
Chikago	3,800	60
Nyandeo	2,400	38
Mkamba A	3,200	50
Mkamba B	2,050	32
Total	11,450	180

made after the pre-test. The interviews were conducted in Swahili. To ensure that all the questionnaires had been properly filled in, one of the enumerators and the researcher, daily checked all the questionnaires. Themes explored in the survey included:

- Household socio-economic and demographic characteristics (age, sex, level of education, headship, occupation, household members relation to the household head, in/out migration, deaths experienced over the past five to ten years, duration of residence and income).
- Health status (short, chronic and prolonged sickness of household members).
- Livelihood activities and assets (on farm, off-farm and non-farm activities; amount and size of assets).
- Food security strategies (own production of food, purchase, food exchange, food help and claims; and food insecurity coping mechanisms).
- Social capital:
  - Reciprocal relations (engagement in mutual help, giving or receiving support, number and type of people one can call upon in case of need).
  - Membership in formal groups (members and non-members).
  - Involvement in communal/voluntary activities.
  - Experiences with behaviours requiring trust.
  - Expectations of benefits or participation in community collective actions.

Most of the items in the questionnaire, especially those considered sensitive such as food status or health status, were cross-checked by asking the same question in different ways.

vi. Group inventory

This method helped in the identification of formal groups which people are involved in. Group leaders from the groups the respondents mentioned that they were members of during the household survey were interviewed. Group leaders were asked about different aspects, such as total number of members, group diversity in terms of gender, socio-economic status of members, conditions for membership, links with other groups in the area or outside, expected benefits and obligations of group members. The groups from which group leaders interviewed came from are women's groups, and saving-and-credit, religious, tribal, neighbourhood, and producers groups.

vii. The case study, life history and genealogical method

The case study method is used when 'how' or 'why' questions are explored and when the focus is on phenomena that are occurring within real life contexts (Yin, 2003). This method was used to obtain information on the critical life experiences of individuals in the households so as to understand changes over time in their lives. It facilitated studying the changes, dynamics and the problems of coping with insecurities in daily life. This method made possible the follow-up on the important daily events of these households, and revealed how families generate their livelihood and how they cope with prolonged illness, death and food insecurity. In-depth case studies facilitated studying events or phenomena and interrelationship through time. Using a loosely structured interview checklist, life histories addressed important questions on migration history, occupational history, coping mechanisms and mutual sharing activities. Such information helped to reconstruct how households had responded to insecurities in the past. The in-depth interviewing in the framework of applying the case study method also allows for revealing people's own perceptions and how they experience their situation.

After the survey, a preliminary analysis was done to classify households according to different characteristics. With the help of the research assistants, 15 cases were selected for in-depth study, based on the following criteria:

- HIV/AIDS status (affected and non-affected).
- Headship (male-headed and female-headed).
- Resource and assets ownership (well-off and poor).

The genealogical method was used to map the kinship network, to determine the quality and quantity of support one gets from kin and how this is affected by AIDS, because of the reduction of the number relatives who could be a source of support in times of need. In-depth case studies through ego-centric analysis provided a framework for studying social networks, labour relations, and social interaction. Since the social relations of a household and its access to interpersonal support from kin, friends and neighbours are mostly likely to be maintained by women, women provide a good entry point for analysis. It has been widely documented that women are more likely to engage in informal interactions (see Chapter 2). Principal care-givers and or heads of the household were asked to name people on whom they rely for material and non-material help. The focus here was on the type, strength and direction of relationships within networks. To be able to distinguish the effects of HIV/AIDS on social networks and support from other effects, this study compared affected households and non-affected households. Table 3.4 presents the 15 households selected as case studies, their characteristics and the themes they represent. Out of 15 cases, two were orphans, seven had persons who were ill, three experienced death of one or more household members, and three were non-HIV/AIDS-affected.

Table 3.4. Summary of case studies' characteristics and themes they represent.

Case number[a]	Characteristics	Themes
5.1: Naomi	Double-orphaned girl	Loss of skills, change in livelihood activities, lack of kinship support, changes in social norms
5.2: Castor	Paternal orphan boy	Children-headed household, food insecure, inability to cope
5.3: Mama Mkago	De-facto female-headed, poor with 4 orphans, HIV/AIDS-affected.	Caring for orphans
5.4: Mama Oliva	Female-headed Widow, poor, HIV/AIDS-affected	Caring for AIDS patient, changes in livelihood activities
5.5: Mama Zalima	Female-headed, poor, HIV/AIDS-affected	Food insecurity
5.6: Hawa	Well-off, HIV/AIDS-affected, polygamous	Coping sustainably with AIDS
5.7: Mr. Kanyango	Poor, male-headed, polygamous, HIV/AIDS-affected	Inability to cope with AIDS impacts, gender relations
5.8: Mama Wawili	Poor, non-HIV/AIDS-affected, female-headed	Livelihood vulnerability
5.9: Zakia	Young, poor and food insecure	Effects of distant farming
6.1: Mama Dorothy	Female-headed divorced, poor, HIV/AIDS-affected	Lack of kinship support
6.2: Mzee Manda	Elderly household, poor HIV/AIDS-affected	Urban-rural migration of AIDS patients, loss of remittances
6.3: Mama James	Food insecure, HIV/AIDS-affected, deserted by her husband, critically ill	Support from neighbours and friends, food insecurity, lack of family support
6.4: Mama Kandoro	HIV/AIDS-affected, poor	Witchcraft, lack of family support
7.1: Mama Maiko	Well-off, male-headed household, non-HIV/AIDS-affected	Group membership
7.2: Mr. Mlogola	Poor, HIV/AIDS-affected	Non-group membership, HIV/AIDS-affected, stigma

[a] The numbers correspond to the order and the chapters in which they are presented.

viii. Participant observation

Participant observation was one of the main tools used throughout the study. The method allows researchers to immerse themselves in the day to day activities of the people whom they are attempting to understand (May, 1997; Bernard, 2002). It includes more than looking, listening and experiencing and requires living in the area for some time so as to establish and maintain relationships with the people being studied. The method was used to collect data on what actually people do, because people do not always do what they say they (should or intend to) do. Therefore, observation was focused on actual household activities and people's behaviours. The method enabled the researcher to examine the effects and dynamics of social arrangements in informal and formal networks and to see how people recourse to these networks to cope with insecurities. Support during funerals and weddings, labour sharing and food assistance were observed, as well as care activities such as feeding and nursing patients. Other aspects observed included division of labour by gender and age groups, engagement in various livelihood activities, participation in groups and communal activities.

3.5.2 Recruitment of research assistants

Being new in the area, there was a need of having assistants to introduce me and help organize many of the activities related to the fieldwork. Assistants were recruited from the village, since they knew the area and the people. Selection of field assistants was based on gender, influence and personality. A friendly personality was deemed important for enlisting the cooperation of the community members during the study. One man and one woman were recruited as field assistants, who later were immersed in the study after a series of meetings with a researcher and participating in most of the initial contacts the researcher had with different individuals, households and groups. They facilitated the focus group discussions and were responsible for logistical arrangements of the various meetings the researcher had in the village.

Enumerators were recruited to assist in the household survey. These were experienced people who had been involved in a number of national and local surveys in and out of Morogoro region. They were recruited from outside the community and were trained prior to the questionnaire pre-test. The training emphasized the main objectives of the study and how concepts used in the study were operationalized. It was vital to get people from outside the research area, since respondents would have not felt at ease to discuss sensitive issues with people they already knew, for fear of their situation becoming known to fellow community members.

3.5.3 Secondary data collection

Secondary sources consisting of records and documented reports contained useful information for this study. These sources enabled me to get general information on demographic facts and on livelihoods and developments during the past five to ten years to provide a historical context for the study's findings. The information was obtained from different government offices and NGOs in the area. Documents, written reports and secondary information related to intra- and inter-household relations and livelihoods were also gathered. Other sources included ethnographic reports, household budget surveys, household census, livelihood survey reports and regional HIV/AIDS reports.

3.6 Data analysis

Quantitative data collected were subjected to bivariate and multivariate analysis. Composite variables were created to determine a household's socio-economic and food security status and the strength of its informal social network. The creation of composite variables and their categorization were done to characterize households in a more comprehensive manner and manage the data easily.

A food security status index was constructed by combining responses from questions on:
- consumption of less preferred food;
- reducing food quantities;
- borrowing either food or money to buy food;
- skipping a meal in a day;
- skipping meals for the whole day.

The five items were scored as follows: 1 = often, 2 = one to four times, 3 = never. They were the combined to form a food security scale, yielding a Cronbach's alpha of 0.84 (cf. Field, 2005). Households were categorized based on the number of times they reported to have applied food insecurity responses. A maximum score of fifteen indicates that the household has never applied coping responses and can therefore be considered to be food secure. A score between eleven and fourteen indicates moderate food insecurity, meaning that these households have used coping responses from time to time. A score between five and ten indicates a food-insecure status.

An informal social network scale was constructed from responses to three items from the household survey questionnaire, which are:
- The number of people willing to help in case of food shortage.
- The number of people willing to help in case of prolonged illness.

- The number of people who have turned to the respondent for help during the three months prior to the interview.

The three items were scored as follows: 1 = no one; 2 = one to four people; 3 = five or more people. They were combined to form a homogeneous informal social network scale (Cronbach's alpha 0.61). The total score for informal social capital ranged from three to nine, yielding three groups of households with low (score 3 to 4), moderate (score 5 to 7), and high informal social capital (score 8 to 9), respectively.

The socio-economic status of households was measured by combining eight questionnaire items to provide a score to rank households as poor (low score) to well-off (high score) status. These included:

- House ownership.
- Quality of the house (1 = good condition, 0 = bad condition).
- Land ownership.
- TV ownership.
- Bike ownership.
- Mobile phone ownership.
- Livestock ownership.

The items on ownership were scored 1 for owning and 0 for not-owning. The items were combined to form a socio-economic status scale (Cronbach's alpha 0.59). The values ranged from a minimum of zero to a maximum of seven, with 0 to 2 being poor, 3 to 4 being moderately poor and 5 to 7 well-off.

Qualitative data from the focus group discussions, case studies, life histories, and key-informant interviews were interpreted and organized into different themes based on conceptual description of ideas as expressed by the respondents during the interviews and focus group discussions. These themes were then related to the study questions. Extracts of interview transcripts from case studies, comment or clusters of comments from the key informant interviews and focus group discussions in relation to the issues investigated are presented in the following chapters.

3.7 Validity and reliability

Validity and reliability are vital methodological concepts for designing and implementing rigorous and high-quality qualitative and quantitative research. Validity is defined as the degree to which one measures what one is supposed to measure. In scientific research, appropriateness and accuracy of measurement are of great importance. The reliability of a research instrument concerns the extent to which the instrument yields the same results on repeated trials. Because they yield 'rich' descriptive data, qualitative research methods enable an in-depth understanding of the phenomena concerned. However, such findings usually fail to give an indication of the level of prevalence and the distribution of such phenomena. They may also suffer from researcher's subjectivity, which may detrimental to the study. The power of the qualitative methods lies in their ability to address validity concerns. By trying to get a deeper understanding of phenomena, it is easy to assess whether they are capturing the essence of phenomena that are being measured. Qualitative research designs are associated with interpretative approaches, capturing the informants' emic point of view, rather than measuring discrete, observable behaviour. Contrary to qualitative research methods, Creswell (1998:15) described quantitative research as 'an inquiry based on testing a theory composed of variables measured with numbers and analyzed in statistical procedures in order to determine whether the predictive generalization of the theory hold true'. When compared with qualitative methods, the weakness of quantitative research designs lies mainly in their failure to elicit underlying meanings and motivations, their strength in generalization and amenability to statistical testing of distribution patterns.

Although the nature of these two approaches differs and both have their strengths and limitations, their ultimate purpose is the same, which is to obtain an understanding of the phenomena in question. This study aimed at achieving a situation where blending qualitative and quantitative methods of research would yield a final product that could highlight the significant contributions of both methods. Triangulation was used to improve validity of study findings. It was done according to data source (i.e. gathering the same information from various individuals) and method (i.e. qualitative and quantitative). Linking information from both methods and all sources helped to explain the meaning of different phenomena as well as explaining some of the gaps. Repeated visiting by the researcher in the course of applying the qualitative methods enhanced validity. Reliability was ensured by using structured questionnaires and checklists of issues to be discussed with key informants as well as by careful training of field assistants who took part in the household survey. The study also drew information and data from the literature to validate some of the findings. In case the findings were not corresponding with previous research, detailed account is given on such divergences.

3.8 Discrepancies and methodological problems

In research, selection and measurement biases are methodological concerns which researchers strive to minimize but are sometimes unavoidable. These biases could have been introduced during the selection of research units and during the measurement of variables in the study. Obtaining accurate responses is challenging in all research involving human beings (Sharon, 1999). Depending on the subject matter people may not always tell the truth. Obtaining truthful responses was a particular challenge since this study involved exploring sensitive issues such as HIV/AIDS, gender relations and food security. Many respondents did not disclose their HIV/AIDS status for fear of loosing their social reputation or because they consider such information to be private. There were occasional mismatches between how individual respondents answered the questions on food security in the survey and the information gathered from focus group discussions and case studies. It was also observed that respondents tended to give normative answers, especially to questions about support from their social networks and about food insecurity, meaning that especially on these two topics there was a tendency to present a more positive picture than the actual situation allowed. In other instances people responded to what they thought the interviewer wanted to hear or what they thought would impress the interviewer. Some of the questions required people to recall what happened in the past months, which sometimes was difficult for people to recollect exactly and the time lapse affected the reliability of their answers. As a result of such discrepancies, there were inconsistencies between household survey responses and those collected from key informants, case studies and focus group discussions. Nevertheless, these limitations were dealt with by collecting and comparing the same information from various sources. Repeated visits to the same subjects enabled probing and cross-checking of responses given with respect to a particular case. However, despite efforts to resolve these methodological problems, caution is needed when interpreting the results. In cases where this applies, it is highlighted in the discussion of the results.

3.9 Ethical considerations

Informed consent is a vital aspect of research. It is essential to ensure that people involved in the study understand the negative as well as positive consequences of their participation in the research process. To ensure this, I applied for a research permit from Tanzania Council for Science and Technology, which was then presented to the district authority, who gave me a formal letter to work in the village. In preliminary meetings with the village authorities the aims and set-up of the research were introduced. Participation in the study was entirely voluntarily. As said, anonymity and confidentiality are very important for sensitive topics like HIV/AIDS. The questionnaires and cases were named for easy identification and follow-up but this information was not disclosed to anybody except for the data entry assistant and supervisors. In this publication the names of those who took part in the study are pseudonyms, to safeguard anonymity and confidentiality. The respondents in the survey and other persons interviewed were assured that their answers would be treated confidentially.

3.10 Time schedule of the research

i. Phase one: April 2003 – April 2004

This period was spent attending courses necessary for meeting the academic qualifications of the Mansholt Graduate School for Social Sciences, but also courses useful for the research problem articulation. Intensive literature search and synthesis and proposal writing was completed this phase in the Netherlands. In December 2003 a reconnaissance visit to the research area was made to gain more information about the research area. Then finalization of the research proposal was done back in the Netherlands.

ii. Phase two: May 2004 – August 2005

During this period the fieldwork in Tanzania was conducted. It started by processing of the research permit and recruitment of fieldwork assistants. Relevant secondary information was collected from various sources such as district and village offices, the statistics bureau, libraries, national and international organizations and research centres. Qualitative information was gathered from individual key informants and from the focus group discussions. Later the questionnaires were designed and administered to the selected sample. Preliminary analysis of the survey results led to the selection of case studies involved in in-depth interview, life histories, genealogies and egocentric network analysis.

The fieldwork was divided into three stages (see Table 3.5). Stage one used qualitative methods such as participant observation, open-ended interviews with key informants as well as focus group discussions. This formed the explorative phase of the fieldwork. It was meant to elicit patterns related to the research questions as well as for further operationalization of the concepts. The second stage involved sampling of households, household survey and group inventories. Preliminary analysis of the results of the household survey enabled the selection of the cases to include in the in-depth study. Stage three involved in-depth interviews with case study, life histories and discussions on the emerging important features and trends from the survey.

iii. Phase three: September 2005 – April 2007

Thesis write-up - detailed work on the theoretical concepts used in the study; data analysis and description of the study findings and conclusions were done during this phase.

iv. Phase four: May-December 2007

Finalization and English editing of the thesis, and defense.

Table 3.5. Stages and time frame of the fieldwork.

Activity	2004							2005						
	J	J	A	S	O	N	D	J	F	M	A	M	J	J
Organizing research permits and preliminary visit to the area and observation	■													
Collection of secondary data for the previous 5-10 years	■	■												
Exploratory research with key informants and FGDs			■	■	■									
Developing questionnaires					■	■								
Training enumerators							■							
Pre-testing								■						
Household survey								■	■					
Groups inventory								■	■					
Data entry and preliminary data analysis and interpretation										■	■			
Selection of sub-sample for in-depth study												■	■	■
In-depth case study interviews and life histories												■	■	■
Verifying, collecting missing or additional data														■

Chapter 4

Study area and context

This chapter sketches the socio-economic environment of the study area and of the households therein. It presents a picture of how these households are organized and people arrange their livelihoods in the context of a changing environment. The specific features of Mkamba village, on which the research was focused, are described to place the data in context. The complexity and diversity of rural livelihoods include a range of responses to shocks and stresses. HIV/AIDS is one among the shocks affecting people in the area although there are efforts to control the situation. The chapter starts with presenting an overview of the provision of basic health and HIV/AIDS services in Tanzania, followed by a description of the situation with respect to HIV/AIDS in the Morogoro region of which the study area is a part. Subsequently, a short description of Kilombero district is provided and the history of the settlement patterns in the area is discussed, after which the chapter zooms in on Mkamba village and the cultural practices and livelihood activities found there. The sugarcane plantation in the area receives specific attention because of its profound impacts on livelihoods in Mkamba.

4.1 Basic health and HIV/AIDS services in Tanzania

Soon after independence the Government of Tanzania opted for a health policy that aimed at providing a health service to all Tanzanians free of charge. Numerous health facilities were constructed, mainly in rural areas, and staffs were trained to work in these facilities. Tanzania also opted for primary health care in 1978 as an approach to achieve the goal of health for all by 2000. However, this expansion proved to be beyond the management capacity of the government. Being the sole provider of health services, the burden became too heavy for the government (Tarimo *et al.*, 2003). Due to poor national economic performance, the escalating costs of public health care service provision, the emergence of pandemic diseases such as HIV/AIDS and changes in patterns of other diseases, the government's ability to continue providing free health services to all citizens was curtailed (Mubyazi *et al.*, 2000). Government investments in the health sector declined, leading to deteriorating conditions of health facilities, shortage of drugs and other medical supplies, and low staff morale.

These conditions necessitated changes so as to improve the health sector in Tanzania. Health sector reforms took place by redefining the role of the state, decentralisation of health services to local authorities, and enhancing the role of other actors and the private sector in the delivery of goods and services. At the national level the

Ministry of Health is responsible for improving the capacity for sector management, policy development, analysis and national planning, development of guidelines for national policy implementation, performance monitoring, evaluation, legislation, and regulation of service delivery and practice (MOH, 1999). Though most of the health programs and activities are implemented at district level, overall monitoring and supervision is done at regional level. Health reforms have resulted in the decentralization of health care services, which give more power to the district authority to perform a key role in the implementation of health programs, including the running of health centres and dispensaries in the district. The local government is responsible for drugs and medical supplies procurement, salaries, and staff training and development. It gets funds from the central government, from their own revenue sources and donors as well as from the community through user fees and the community health fund. With these new roles, the district becomes an important actor in the delivery of health care services in the country. However, local authorities are faced with management problems due to the lack of clear roles and responsibilities of the parties involved. They are not trained in drafting development plans and lack the resources (technical and financial) necessary for the implementation of health programs in their districts. As a result health care services have been poorly supported and financed.

Reforms are aiming at improving equity and quality of health care, involving different stakeholders such as the central and local government, development partners, donors, NGOs, CBOs, faith-based health service providers, pharmacies, private hospitals and practitioners, traditional healers and village health workers. The private sector is now seen as a partner rather than an opponent, complementing government health provision and widening consumer choices (Tarimo *et al.,* 2003). Reforms were also about diversification of health financing options. In 1993 a user fee was introduced in the form of cost sharing in all tertiary and referral hospitals. According to the Ministry of Health's policy agenda, cost sharing was to be extended to health centres and dispensaries, so that the communities would participate in financing their health care needs through formal and informal risk pooling mechanisms (MOH, 1996). The government introduced the national health scheme to employees in the formal sector and facilitated the introduction of community health funds in districts to provide opportunities for people in the informal sector to pre-pay their medical care at the time they are able and willing to do so, thus providing secure access to health facilities throughout the year. Households unwilling or unable to do this would be required to pay a fee for use of the facility. Though the user fee and community health fund increased the resources for health services, the numbers of subscribers to community health funds are declining, due to the inability to pay and dissatisfaction for the care quality provided (Munishi, 2003).

Many observers have noted that many poor households are unable to pay user fees. The situation is even worse when it comes to women's accessibility to the health care services. Coupled with poverty, women face social and physical barriers to access health care services. For a woman living in poverty, the user fee has a direct effect on her ability to pay for health care. While women struggle to make their household's ends meet, they have very little left for their own health care. In some cases they make a trade-off not to seek health care in order to be able to meet household needs, such as those for food and other necessities. Sometimes women do not make use of health care because they have no cash income, but it may also be the case that women's health is given low priority (Makundi *et al.*, 2005; Nanda, 2002).

A study on the impact of the user fee for antenatal care in government hospitals in three districts in Tanzania showed a 53.4 percent decline in utilization after the fees were introduced (Hussein & Mujinja, 1997). Another study revealed the same trend (Sahn *et al.*, 2003). When the required payment to the health services increased, the use of the services decreased. Household income is positively associated with health-seeking behaviours (Schellenberg *et al.*, 2003). There is a waiver system to prevent the poorest and other vulnerable groups, such as children under five, pregnant women and the elderly, from loosing access to basic health care. Antenatal care and family planning services are exempted from the user fee. Because of public health considerations, patients with conditions such as AIDS and TBC are exempted, even if they are able to pay. Women form a large proportion of those who are exempted, but most of them do not know they are (Nanda, 2002; Tibandebage & Mackintosh, 2002; Mubyazi *et al.*, 2000). The exemptions are often not well known. Those who know, get their information through informal contacts. In their studies Tarimo *et al.* (2003), Mwisongo *et al.* (2000) and Mubyazi *et al.* (2000) found that people in their study areas were not aware of the exemption for the poor. Though women may be exempted from user fees, there are other costs, for example those related to maternity care, which are relatively high. For poor rural population there are numerous health service costs that individuals or households have to bear even after the payment of user fees. On the other side, there is little incentive for providers to apply exemptions because they need the income from user fees to maintain good quality health care (Nanda, 2002). Rigid payment modalities in public and private hospitals and poor service quality discourage people from seeking treatment from such facilities. Though studies found that user fees contribute to the underutilization of public health facilities, Green (2000) shows that decisions regarding treatment choices depend on how individuals construct the causes of their illness and what they perceive to be quality of the health care provided.

The HIV/AIDS pandemic expanded at the time of economic decline and health sector reforms, posing a threat to further reform initiatives. Dealing with HIV/AIDS requires a multi-sectoral approach to prevent and mitigate its impacts. Such an approach has to combine community-based interventions for prevention and home-based care as well as clinical services for treating STIs, TB and other opportunistic infections and provision of antiretroviral drugs (ARVs). Reduced health-care financing poses threats to the control of and mitigation of HIV/AIDS. AIDS has resulted in massive and mounting demands on already constrained services and resources. Although the country's strategic plan for the health sector in 2003 added another strategy to focus on HIV/AIDS explicitly, there have been few attempts to address simultaneously the problems of the service system and of HIV/AIDS on the basis of a system-wide analysis (Hanson, 2000). HIV/AIDS affects both the human and financial resources on which the health sector reform is based. As AIDS continues to strike, service systems are weakened and fewer resources are available to control the epidemic that has resulted in increased overall mortality. At the same time, health sector reforms sometimes lead to less publicly funded care, which means that a larger burden of unpaid care may fall on women, especially in the context of the HIV/AIDS pandemic. Many of the HIV/AIDS-affected individuals are unable to get proper medical attention for reasons including inability to pay for treatment, poor service delivery, and lack of access to medical facilities and services. While the most critical constraint is a decline in resources, there are also equity issues that arise within the health sector. There is geographical variation in resources distribution which is biased favourably towards urban centres. The districts are constrained in terms of material and human resources to implement HIV/AIDS control programs, despite political commitment.

Following the reforms in the health sector, formal and informal private practitioners have become popular. Many people opt for private health services rather than public ones for various reasons, such as avoiding long waits and perceived good quality of private health care. Alongside formal private practitioners, there are individuals who sell basic health treatments for cash. These are people who have experience in medical work and offer medical services to those who turn to them for help. They are readily available, which makes it convenient to seek their service. There are also voluntary agencies, especially religious organizations, which provide health services to the wider population.

Traditional medicine and practices are recognized in the national health policy. Depending on how they see the cause of their illness, individuals may seek treatment from traditional healers. Traditional healers are consulted when it is felt that the illness cannot be treated in a hospital or is caused by witchcraft or supernatural powers. Although spending on traditional treatment can be as high as and even higher than hospital services, people may still choose traditional therapies. A study in Ifakara, Tanzania, revealed that traditional treatments are flexible and adapted to the economic constraints of the population (Muela *et al.*, 2000). They allow alternatives to cash payments such as payment in kind, in work, or credit. Patients can negotiate the price with the provider. A second payment is required only if the treatment is perceived to be a success. Regardless of where people can be treated, the cost of health care continues to be a significant barrier to service access and use.

In rural areas, there are community-based village health workers who perform community health functions. These health workers are volunteers, who are supposed to be paid by the village authorities. According to the ministry of health structure there should two community-based village health workers per hamlet, who are trained to be able to provide essential health services in the community. Their work includes health education and promotion on environment sanitation, STI/HIV/AIDS issues and family planning, mobilization for immunization, and treating minor ailments. They also do counseling and pay home visits to people with chronic illnesses such as AIDS.

Traditional birth attendants are women who are usually self-taught or informally trained to conduct normal deliveries, provide post-natal care, and advise women on preparation for delivery, attending antenatal care, family planning, STIs and HIV/AIDS. They also refer high-risk pregnant women to the hospital. A TBA may be a full-time worker who can be called upon by anyone and who expects to be paid either in cash or in kind. TBAs are key members of the community who helps women to access necessary service. A study conducted in 47 councils found that among home deliveries, untrained TBAs conducted about 68 percent of deliveries followed by trained TBAs at 18.5 percent and midwives (MCHAs) conducting about 13.7 percent of the total registered deliveries (Makundi *et al.,* 2000). This indicates the importance of TBAs in rural settings.

4.2 The HIV/AIDS situation in Morogoro region

Morogoro region in the south-eastern part of Tanzania has not been spared by the spread of the HIV/AIDS pandemic. AIDS statistics for the region indicate that there has been a rapid increase in HIV/AIDS prevalence among blood donors ranging from zero in 1983 to 20 percent in 2004. Detailed figures for every district from 1999 to 2004 are shown in Table 4.1. High prevalence rates in some years may suggest much voluntary blood donation for the blood transfusion services in the region, because blood donors are tested for HIV and thereby provide a picture of the actual magnitude of the epidemic in the region.

Table 4.1. Morogoro HIV/AIDS prevalence among blood donors 1999-2004.

Year/District	HIV prevalence rate (%)					
	1999	2000	2001	2002	2003	2004
Kilombero	6	16	16	11.5	19	nd
Kilosa	5	16.2	10	6.1	4.7	5.3
Ulanga	6.1	6.4	18	10.6	5.3	4.2
Morogoro Rural	5	11.6	12	nd	7	20.3
Morogoro Urban	8.2	11.9	nd	nd	8.6	7.8

nd - No data.
Source: Regional Health Office - Morogoro.

The number of AIDS cases increased in 2000 (Table 4.2), which could have been caused by a new wave of male migrants coming to work as labourers on the sugar plantations. Data on the new AIDS cases clearly shows the extent of the problem in the region (Table 4.2).

Table 4.2. Reported new AIDS cases by district Morogoro region 1998-2004.

District	Number of new AIDS cases						
	1998	1999	2000	2001	2002	2003	2004
Kilombero	818	684	793	453	nd	310	333
Ulanga	75	39	242	39	nd	177	149
Kilosa	91	78	308	142	nd	57	59
Morogoro Rural	90	138	181	168	nd	53	176
Morogoro Urban	700	626	778	749	nd	394	273
Total	1774	1565	2302	1551	nd	991	990

nd- No data.
Source: Regional Health Office - Morogoro.

4.3 Kilombero District

Kilombero is one of the districts in the Morogoro region situated in the flood plains of the Kilombero River, which extends 250 kilometres from Southwest to Northwest. The district is bordered by the Udzungwa range of mountains in the Northeast and Mahenge Mountains in the Southwest. In Kilombero, agriculture accounts for about 80 percent of the district's income (Kilombero District Development Plan, 2003). Most villagers grow rice, maize and cassava for household consumption. Production of rice and maize also caters for household cash flow. Maize and rice are usually sold to private buyers who trade in the local market and also sell to other regions of Tanzania. Households utilize family labour and in a few cases hired labour. Other activities include fishing, small-scale trading, and nomadic pastoralism. Some men earn an additional income as casual labourers and fishermen. Women sell farm produce and their labour to earn cash.

The kinship system among the ethnic groups in the area is mainly patrilineal. This has implications for access to land, household labour organization and rights over property. Kilombero district is characterized by a remarkable ethnic heterogeneity. It is not uncommon to find members of several different ethnic groups in one village, like in the research village. The heterogeneity is due to in-migration mainly caused by the villagization policy of the early 1970s and employment opportunities in the district. The ethnic groups, locally referred to as indigenous people, comprise the Wamdamba, Wambunga and Wapogoro, who arrived in the early 19th century from Malawi and the Southern part of Tanzania. The Wandamba are closely related to Wapogoro, who occupy the western part of the valley basin and the adjacent Mahenge Highlands. Other tribes that migrated to the Kilombero Valley include the Wasagara, Wahehe, Wabena, Wandendeule, Wasukuma, Wangoni, Wangindo, Wamang'ati, and Wachaga, to mention a few. The construction of TAZARA railway in 1972 brought an influx of other ethnic groups from different parts of the country, such as Wanyakyusa, Wandali, Wakinga and Wakisi to the valley. Swahili is the lingua franca, but in daily life people speak their own language.

The figures in Tables 4.1 and 4.2 indicate that Kilombero district has been greatly hit. Poverty is noted to be a main factor contributing to the spread of HIV/AIDS in Kilombero (ESRF, 2005). Mobility has been associated with increasing risk to HIV infection. The concentration of male migrants isolated from their families increases the demand for commercial sex, which facilitates the spread of HIV. Kilombero attracts a so-called 'mobile population', which consist of people who stay away from home for varied periods of time during a year. They are at both risk of HIV-infection and are contributing to the spread of the virus. They include traders, migrant farmers, casual/seasonal labourers and truck drivers. Their comparative wealth enables them to engage in paid sex. Since most of the people in the area are predominantly poor, engagement in transactional sex is one of the surviving strategies (ESRF, 2005), and in so doing many are exposed to HIV. Many of the seasonal casual labourers recruited to work in sugar cane plantations come from highly affected regions in Tanzania, such as Mbeya and Iringa. If affected, their movement to Kilombero may result in further spread of HIV. They may also get infected in the area of destination. The direction of infection is not only from mobile men to local women but also vice versa. Inability to negotiate safe sex and unprotected sexual practices among mobile population groups, involving multiple partners, make people susceptible to HIV infection. It has been found that among farm and plantation workers in Iringa and Morogoro, for example, HIV-prevalence is about 30 percent, (cf. Tanzania national website accessed on 30/08/07) which is high compared to the general population (7%).

Guided by the National Multi-Sectoral Framework (NMSF) the district has a HIV/AIDS plan to prevent new infections and mitigate HIV/AIDS impacts. There are significant interventions involving different stakeholders such as the local government, communities, CBOs and NGOs. The interventions include condom distribution, conducting seminars to reduce stigma and discrimination and create awareness on prevention, helping the community to eradicate harmful practices, sensitization for voluntary counseling and testing, research and disseminating essential information on HIV/AIDS. Ireland Aid and UNICEF have facilitated the establishment of school and out-of-school clubs and training of peer educators to make the community aware of HIV/AIDS and related problems. Such groups also point to risky traditions and beliefs, like female genital mutilation, widow inheritance and the *nyasika* custom (staying with one's daughter as a temporal spouse). The organization AXIOS is supporting the Prevention of Mother-to-Child Transmission (PMCTC) program, which started in September 2003 and is now operating in 26 antenatal centres in the district, including the Mkamba dispensary. An increased number of volunteers are joining the PMCTC program. Since its establishment, about 3,150 women have been counseled, of whom 2,505 were willing to undergo an HIV-test and 175 were found to be HIV-affected (District Report, 2004). There is also an organization of people-living-with HIV/AIDS (SHDEPHA^{+}) at district level, dedicated to care and support, and treatment of opportunistic infections of individuals living with HIV/AIDS. Among the common diseases in Kilombero is malaria which is known to interact with HIV (Corbett, 2002). Malaria was identified as a major public health problem in Kilombero valley, which contributes to a considerable burden with premature deaths and disability from illness (Tarner *et al.*, 1991).

4.4 Settlement patterns and village governance in Tanzania

Rural life in Tanzania has been profoundly influenced by colonial rule and post-colonial efforts to improve the lives of the people. During the German period, the population was scattered into small settlements spread over a wide area. The Germans recognized the difficulty of controlling a dispersed population. When the British came, they implemented a close settlement policy to facilitate state control. In the late 1950s the British colonial administrators initiated what they called 'the community development approach' for rural transformation. This program was implemented through resettlement of farmers into closely supervised communities so that extension services could easily reach them. After Independence, in 1961, the new government also embarked upon a rural improvement and transformation program to increase and modernize agricultural production. This program worked along the existing policy of farmers' assistance that aimed at helping progressive farmers to increase their agricultural output. It basically consisted of efforts to gradually raise output among rural households through extension services.

The transformation sought to radically transform agriculture through the resettlement in special schemes of pre-selected villagers who would then engage in modern farming under the supervision and direction of state officials. The settlers were provided with infrastructures and inputs to improve agricultural production. By the end of 1965 there were 23 such schemes with some 15,000 acres of crops and about 3,400 farming families (Mapolu, 1990). By 1966, however, it became clear that the 'improvement' approach was not producing substantial results. Although the area under cash crops production increased over the years, output continued to fluctuate as a result of climatic conditions and increased input prices. As for the 'transformation' approach, government soon realized it was incurring enormous costs to establish and run the settlement schemes whose production continued to be minimal. It emerged that the resettled farmers tended to see themselves as government employees rather as than independent farmers receiving government technical assistance (Mapolu, 1990). The program failed due to heavy costs and because such a program could not be run without foreign assistance. Under this program people were moved from semi-arid areas to the fertile areas of Pangani/Wami basin and the Kilombero river basin. This movement may also have been a factor in the ethnic diversity of Kilombero district.

Later on, Tanzania firmly committed itself to building an egalitarian society through socialism and self-reliance, as outlined in the Arusha Declaration of 1967. In the early 1970's, the social engineering project to build communal villages called *Vijiji vya Ujamaa* (Ujamaa villages) brought scattered inhabitants from remote areas to organized villages. These settlement schemes were rooted in the colonial community development approach. But learning from the past settlement program, villages that were established after the Arusha declaration had to rely on their own developmental resources. To improve the socio-economic position of many Tanzanians, and guided by socialist ideology, people were forced to live in *Ujamaa* villages. The assumptions behind the formation of Ujamaa villages were based on the traditional family values of mutual respect, sharing of basic goods and services and the obligation of everybody to work. Ideally, a village was envisaged to have a primary school, a dispensary, and a clean water supply. The consequences of the resettlement of the rural population into model villages have been the subject of heated debate. It has been argued that villages are successful as organizational units for government services but not as organizational public production units. In some areas agricultural collectivization was imposed. Villages created as part of the *Ujamaa* drive were to function as economic units producing surplus on a communal plot. Villagization was expected to facilitate the provision of public services, but also to allow the possibility of large-scale farming.

In Tanzania, the villagization program was implemented irrespective of its consequences for agriculture - an occupation which most of those affected relied on. By 1979 a total of 8,200 villages were established, involving about 87 percent of the rural population (Sendaro, 1991). Farming was largely affected, because since there was no formal reorganization of land allocation, most people continued to farm on their own plots. The households' increased distance from their farms posed a major problem. It resulted in split residence with people officially living in the formally recognized village while at the same time spending much of the agricultural year in temporal houses and shelters on their old farms. Because of this, villagization scattered families over villages. The state input delivery system associated with villagization affected agricultural production. Untimely delivery and poor storage of inputs reduced input's efficiency. Likewise the use of modern inputs required additional labour while villagization had caused labour shortages. People were moved into areas where the population density was already high, which made it difficult for them to get basic services and farming plots. Among other factors, the decline and stagnation of the country's agricultural productivity from mid-1970s to mid-1980s is partly attributed to the effects of villagization policy (Skarstein, 2005). People were settled on land belonging to other villagers, which led to conflicts over the existing and uncultivated lands. Community divisions in villages were historically formed along ethnic or religious lines. During this time, however, because of new relations that emerged and the inability of the government to provide for the newcomers, an economic crisis developed and the number of witchcraft accusations rose in most of the villages involved (Stroeken, 2001; Mesaki, 1994). Believed to be inspired by the jealousy of neighbours who seemed to be surpassing the rest of the community in financial and material gains, witchcraft accusations became rampant in these villages. Societal divisions, witchcraft and the failures of villagization still dominate people's minds, which may be partly responsible for current low level of community trust and lack of communal initiatives.

Migration of people within and even among countries in search for employment is of all times and is by no means a new phenomenon in Tanzania. Prior to colonisation population movements were associated with warfare, natural calamities and the search for fertile land, but this was essentially rural to rural migration (Liviga & Mekacha, 1998). Migration became common during the German and British colonial periods in the wake of an export-oriented economy and an emphasis on urban sector development (Mwalimu, 2004). Colonial economic systems of labour reserve and the settlers' plantations resulted in the movement of labour to the sisal, coffee, cotton and sugar plantations in the country. Areas where colonial regimes did not introduce cash crops plantations became sources of migratory labour. A study conducted by Lazaro (1996) found that sugar and sisal plantations in Morogoro attracted people from different parts of the country and even from other countries like Mozambique, Rwanda and Burundi. This can explain the population diversity in Mkamba village, as people also migrated to this area seeking employment in the sugar cane plantations. A decline in agricultural production in the mid-1980s resulted in declining incomes, which might also have forced people to seek employment in plantations (Mbilinyi, 1997). The construction of the Kidatu hydro-electric power plant in 1969 and its operation to date have entailed employing people from various parts of the country. Also the construction of the TAZARA railway line in 1971 contributed to the influx of different people from different regions of Tanzania currently living in Kilombero district. Both the sugar cane plantations and the hydro-electric power station are partly in Mkamba village, and the TAZARA railway line passes through it.

4.5 Mkamba village

4.5.1 Socio-economic and demographic characteristics

Mkamba village is sandwiched between the Kilombero sugar plantations to the East and Udzungwa Mountains National park to the West, Kidatu village to the South and Kilosa district to the North (Figure 4.1). People's settlements are dense and confined by the foot slopes of the mountains and the sugar plantation plains. The history of Mkamba village can be traced back to the colonial periods. Mkamba village was named after a man who was a leader of a group called Wamawanda. In 1942 there was an operation of moving people from across the Ruaha River to the Mkamba area. The Wamawanda came with their leader, formerly called *Jumbe*, now

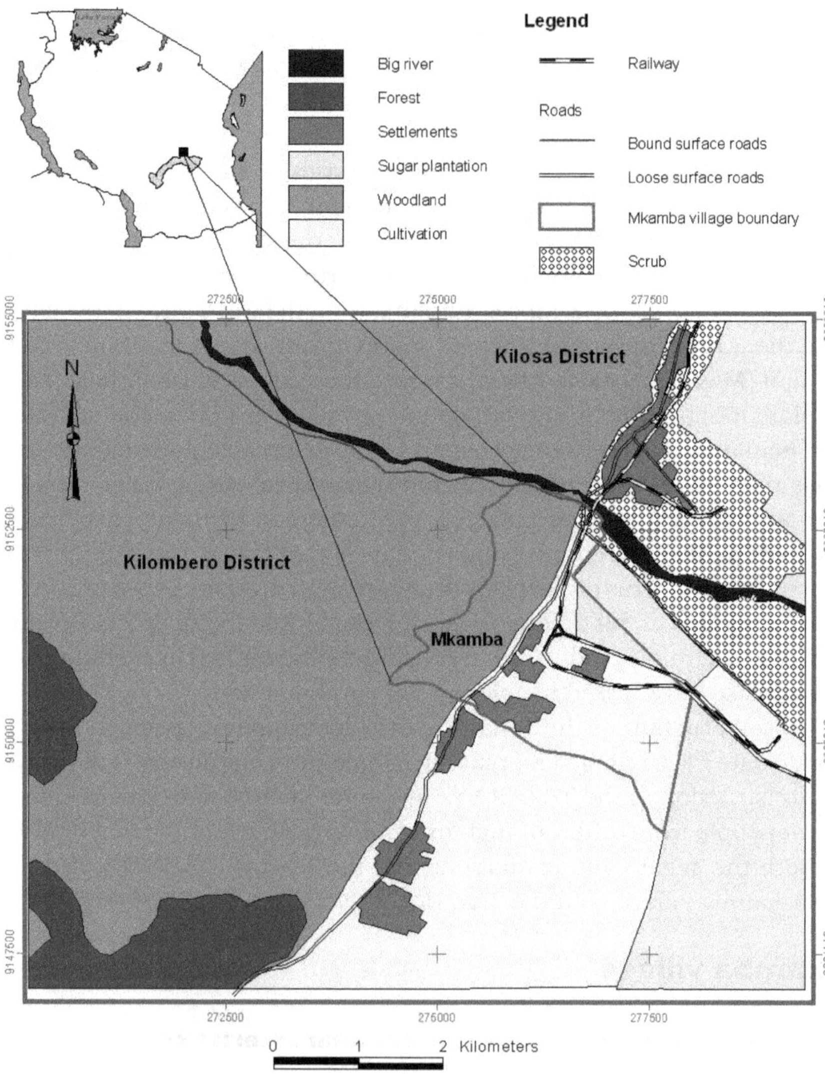

Figure 4.1. Mkamba village map.

Balozi (a 10-cell leader[2]). Since the area was too big for the existing leader to rule, Jumbe Mkamba was given the area which the village occupies now. This movement brought in other ethnic groups from Morogoro region, such as the Wasagala, Waluguru

[2] These are unpaid ruling party officials, either men or women, selected to be responsible for a group of ten households although there might be more than ten households. Their roles are political and administrative, though they are mainly used in settling families' disputes.

and Wavidunda. As one old man recalled, by the year 1957 there were only 48 tax payers. Now, the population has increased tremendously as a result of employment opportunities created by industries and the greater accessibility of the village by the railway. Employment opportunities and easy accessibility to the village has brought people from all corners of Tanzania, resulting in a high degree of ethnic heterogeneity in the village.

Due to urban expansion and the designation of peri-urban or village lands as planning areas (Kironde, 2004), Mkamba was designated as a small town, but at the same time has remained a village under by the 1999 Village Act. By this act, land is owned under customary law, but once areas are declared to be a planning area, customary tenure does no longer apply and the tenure status becomes uncertain. In the village there are plots under customary laws and plots that are legally owned under lease arrangements. This situation poses problems in dealings with land and causes conflicts.

Mkamba is divided into six sub-villages (hamlets), which are divided into 10-cells units. All the village affairs are discussed and decided upon by the village council, which is chaired by the village chairman who can be selected from any political party by the village assembly. The village council is under a chairperson who is assisted by the Village Executive Office (VEO), who is a district employee. There are sub-committees responsible for planning, social services, environmental, and relief issues. Although villages ought to have an HIV/AIDS committee, Mkamba has none. In ordinary planning procedures, new ideas emerge from different planning committees. After thorough discussion they are then put on the agenda of the council meeting. The consensus reached in village assemblies culminates in the identification of key problems and solutions and, ultimately, the formulation of projects. It is important to note here that some of the ideas taken on board by the village councils originate from informal discussions, for example in a local bar, during funerals, etc. In such gatherings, sometimes important issues of concern are raised, discussed and finally taken aboard for further action. Under the political multi-party system, there are five political parties, but only two parties (CCM and CUF) are active in the village. The village council has members from these two parties, which sometimes creates tensions and misunderstanding and, consequently, affects the implementation of the decisions taken. Most of the respondents see the village council as having a great potential as an institutional framework for village governance and development. However, some people commented that the village councils have a poor overall record in the management of community-owned resources.

Although the Sugar Company is autonomous, administratively the people working for the Sugar Company are members of Mkamba village and they form one of the six hamlets with a representative in the village council. They are answerable and report to the village local government as in other villagers. The company is represented by its public relation officer in the security and development committee in the village council. Like other villagers, they are supposed to participate in all village activities such as village meetings and in other public interest activities. For example, in construction work the Company participates by offering machinery for road construction or money for activities which require cash contributions. In case the Company intends to do any development work in the area, it is discussed with the village council. Villagers make use of services provided by the Company such as housing for teachers and health officers, services like hospitals, schools and police. In collaboration with other stakeholders, the company facilitated the establishment of the Kilombero Trust fund in 2005. It undertakes projects to develop out-growers farming activities and uses available funds for the benefit of Kilombero District community. The Sugar Company has invested in social development, schools, hospitals, primary courts and the construction of portable water systems in the district.

The village counted a total population of 12,737 in 2003 (Village Report, 2003), compared to 6,711 people in 1978 (URT, 1978). The total area of the village is estimated to be 6.322 square Kilometers with a population density of 2,014 people per square Kilometers. This is a remarkable figure can be attributed to the fact that many people live in rented rooms since they have no plots or houses of their own in the village. It is quite common to find more than five households living in one house. The population increases during the peak of the sugarcane harvest (May to December) when about 5,000 to 6,000 casual labourers are recruited from other regions. Some of them settle in the village, first living in the estate camps during the sugarcane harvest and then renting rooms in the village. Due to in-migration the Mkamba population is increasing rapidly. Most of the incoming population is being squeezed in the limited public lands in the village. There is no room for extending those because the village is surrounded by sugar cane plantations and protected forest areas.

4.5.2 Basic services

The public dispensary is the first health facility in the community. It forms the backbone of the rural health services that offer a full range of curative and rehabilitative services to individuals and families. Other services include mother-and-child health (MCH), family planning, immunization, and provision of essential drugs and basic equipments. Mkamba village has a public dispensary serving two villages with a total population of about 25,039 people, and two private hospitals, one owned by the Sugar Company. The public dispensary is managed by a clinical worker who diagnoses and treats common diseases and refers serious cases to the nearest hospital. Common diseases in the village are malaria, diarrhea, sexually transmitted diseases, skin diseases, pneumonia and tuberculosis. The dispensary offers MCH services together with voluntary HIV/AIDS counseling and testing (VCT) and prevention of HIV/AIDS mother-to-child transmission (PMCTC). The latter activities started in September 2003. Like many rural dispensaries, the Mkamba dispensary is mostly lacking in drugs and other supplies, leading to poor services. Despite paying user fees, people complain that there is no improved quality of services in return. Because of this people perceive the public health service to be of low quality, which contributes to their reluctance to make use of such facilities.

The Mkamba dispensary runs a home-based care program for those with prolonged illnesses such as AIDS-related infections, leprosy, and mental problems, together with the community based village health workers. The program is always short of important medicines. Most HIV/AIDS-affected households are not reached because they are unaware of the availability of the program's services, but also because of the secrecy that surrounds HIV/AIDS in the area and people's reluctance to disclose their status.

There has been an increase in traditional healers in Mkamba village, which the people in the village attribute to the increase of prolonged and incurable infections. However, some people are skeptical about the trustworthiness of traditional healers. It was said during the focus group discussions that there are some who cheat and manipulate their patients to obtain money. Traditional birth attendants are also present in Mkamba village and are well integrated in the government health system. Some of them have been trained on maternal health and HIV/AIDS aspects. Their payment varies from recognition to in-kind gifts and modest cash payments.

There are three primary schools in the village plus another two in the sugar factory and TANESCO compounds. The latter are mainly for the children of the employees working in these institutions. The village is well provided with tap water, having water points in several places in the village. Water is tapped from the neighbouring Udzungwa Mountains National park and the villagers have a committee coordinated by IKERA that is responsible for system maintenance and levy collection from the households in the village. Maintenance of the water points in different areas in the village is done by the neighbourhood groups and coordinated by ten-cell leaders. These groups made up of ten households are responsible for cleaning and contributing labour for maintenance. Each household pays a monthly contribution for water services.

4.5.3 Households in Mkamba village

The Swahili word for household is *kaya*, which is used in Mkamba as well. Most of the household in Mkamba are male-headed though there are several female-headed households (21% in the sample). Households become female-headed as a consequence of divorce, separation, or death of the partner probably due to AIDS. According to the participants of Focus Group 4 (see Table 3.2) broken marriages are mostly caused by violence, unfaithfulness and alcoholism. Many men who were breadwinners faced lay-off from their job due to large scale privatization in 1998. Some unemployed men in the area could no longer generate enough income and deserted their families. There are both *de jure* and *de facto* female household heads. Divorced or separated women tend to remarry, sometimes regardless of the cause of the first marital dissolution. If the former partner was HIV-infected, upon remarriage the new partner will be infected too. Since people do not disclose the cause of death or reasons for divorce or separation, there is a chance to marry an already infected man or woman, thereby increasing the spread of HIV. People tend to determine the health of a new partner by his/her appearance, although this person may be infected by HIV. Polygamy is common, especially among Muslims (36% in the sample). Non-Muslims may have extra marital affairs that are not officially or customarily recognized, which is locally referred to as having 'small houses'.

Conventional definitions of the household emphasize co-residence as key attribute of the household. However, since migration has become a very common phenomenon, household members are not necessarily permanently in one residence but may be spread over different locations at different times. This is also the case with some households in Mkamba. Furthermore, households are not homogeneous; they differ in composition according to gender and age. During the focus group discussions on major problems in the area (FGD 1 and 2, see Table 3.2) it was said that before AIDS most deaths occurred among infants, young children and the elderly. Because of HIV/AIDS morbidity and mortality young adults are dying. Survivors, usually young children and elderly, form new households that show a different composition compared to traditional households.

The division of labour in the research area according to gender presents the following picture. Women perform most of the domestic responsibilities and engage in petty trade activities like food vending, brewing, and sale of charcoal. Most of these activities are home-based. As for farming, both men and women work together on the farm for every operation, like land clearing, ploughing, sowing, weeding and harvesting. Gender differentiation becomes visible after harvest, when men have power to decide how to use the harvest. It is mostly men who are involved in distant travel to market the farm's produce. Both girls and boys participate in farming tasks but girls more than boys do most of the domestic chores. Both young girls and boys hawk items like roasted groundnuts and buns to earn extra income for the household. However, there are gradual changes with regard to division of labour between girls and boys in the household. During focus group discussions, it was said that these days boys also do housework.

4.5.4 Social and community life in the village

Households are related to other households through kinship, neighbourhood groups, gender-based groups, ethnic groups, religious groups, and formal institutions through an array of rights and responsibilities, claims and obligations. Such relations are important for household's livelihood but also as sources of support. The extent to which individuals and household can rely on these networks depends on circumstance and has greatly changed due to various reasons. Moral obligations towards kin are less acknowledged. Most of the exchanges are now mediated by cash. In most informal and formal groups, money contributions have become important, yet most members have problems to make these. Labour exchanges have declined. In the past people used to share labour in activities such as farming, harvesting and house construction, or made local brew and invited other people to work on their plots. Nowadays communal exchanges or sharing are regarded as a thing of the past and out-dated. Local brew or someone's labour is no longer used to secure assistance from kin and neighbours in major undertakings such as harvesting and house construction. A village woman said: 'Nowadays people love money more than relatives, if you have no money, then you are nothing.'

Kinship has always been related to common residence, but due to socio-economic change members of kin groups have become mobile and do not always live nearby. Migration has impacts on the way kinship is organized. It has loosened the links between relatives. In the study area there are many kinship groups belonging to various ethnic groups. Though some kin will be found living in the same area, the kinship support system has been greatly undermined by changing social and economic conditions and cannot be relied upon to provide support for its members. Almost all case studies of HIV/AIDS-affected households revealed[3] that kinship-based arrangements that used to function as a form of social insurance and protect vulnerable family members, have changed. Even though the justification for reciprocal obligations between members of a family is still recognized, implementation is obstructed by economic hardship and self-interest. In the study area, kinship support becomes visible during major life-cycle ceremonies, mainly marriages and deaths. Creighton (1995) noted that there is no life-course rite that brings members of the

[3] The cases concerned are: 5.1, 5.2, 5.3, 5.4, 5.5, 6.1 and 6.3.

kin group together as effectively as funerals. Funerals are also occasions at which non-kinsmen participate voluntarily, but sometimes people participate for fear of being excluded or not helped when faced with the same problem. People realize that deaths in one's family are inevitable and cannot be dealt with without support. Funerals remain the common event that draws people together as a community.

Since relatives are less complying with kinship expectations, in case of problems support can be provided by self-help groups such as ethnic, women and religious groups formed to address different issues in the area. The groups in the community provide support and make available certain material and social resources that their members can access and utilize. In terms of public interest, community members participate in activities such as school construction and maintenance of roads and water points. There are village bylaws that guide participation in communal activities. Those who do not participate without a valid reason are fined. The fines can either be a contribution in kind (labour) or cash to a particular activity. Contributions to communal projects are in kind (labour and locally available materials such as bricks, sand and stones) or in cash. Ten-cell leaders mobilize and coordinate people in their neighbourhood to implement these activities. People participate voluntarily in religious or political activities.

Inter-ethnic relations: Utani

Related to ethnic grouping there are ritual inter-ethnic relationships. There is a special relation among different ethnic groups in Tanzania known as a joking relationship (*utani* in Swahili). Joking relations among ethnic groups have a historical background. Ethnic groups who fought against each other became *watani* (jokers). The practice of *utani* is a unique expression of ancient ethnic rivalries (Booth *et al.,* 1993). Joking relations were developed to ensure sustainability of the peace agreement between the conflicting ethnic groups. The joking relationship is a way to integrate former enemies into one's social group for support. Many ethnic groups in Tanzania claim *utani* relationships to get support in times of funerals or disaster. These relationships used to be very important, much more than they are today and were used to helping each other in accomplishing farming tasks or any other communal activity. Jokers used to be like close relatives, helping in settling conflicts or removing misunderstandings among people from a particular ethnic group. They have certain rules to observe, failure of which will make one of them lose something to his/her *mtani* (singular of *watani*). Joking relationships allow people of different ethnic groups to verbally abuse one another without taking offence. Joking relationships are for both men and women. A woman can joke with a man from another ethnic group and vice versa.

Presently the role of jokers only becomes visible during funerals. The most important rite they perform is the death ceremony and in many cases they act as a close relative during bereavement. Apart from offering emotional support, jokers supervise all burial activities like digging the grave, washing the corpse, bringing in water and firewood, and cooking for the deceased's family and other mourners. Jokers play crucial role in organizing and coordinating funerals, also observing how other community members participate and reporting this to the bereaved family members later on. For example, the female joker identifies the women who come with necessary items required during funerals. Although she may not record their names on paper, she memorizes their names. After burial, jokers are supposed to stay with the relatives of the deceased and do most of the household chores such as cooking and cleaning for the family until the end of mourning period, which used to be forty days. Nowadays, the mourning period has been reduced to a few days, which are only observed by close relatives. In informal interviews and group discussions, people stated that that the joker role is still very important, but also noted that these days jokers in many cases leave the family after the burial. Due to the increased number of deaths and life hardships, it is not possible for them to stay longer because they have to work or attend other funerals.

Witchcraft and cleansing rituals

Witchcraft beliefs and anti-witchcraft initiatives form an important aspect of social life in the study area. A belief in witchcraft allows people to make sense of the arbitrary misfortunes that govern their lives and to pin blame for these events on a particular person rather than on chance (Ashforth, 2001). Witchcraft provides people with explanations for events and circumstances which they would otherwise not be able to explain. According to Golooba-Mutebi (2005) anything that brings about stress and tension among individuals or between groups or even within a community, may spark off a witchcraft accusation. Sources of tension include competition for scarce resources, contrasting social outlooks, joblessness, poverty, drought, illness, and other misfortunes. Mesaki (1994) found that among the Sukuma of Tanzania, a sickness which fails to responds to normal treatment is associated with enmity, envy or jealousy of those with whom the victim interacts. The most significant outcome of the proliferation of witchcraft suspicions and accusations is the negative effect on the way people relate to each other, and many studies tend to overlook the long-term social impacts (Golooba-Mutebi, 2003).

In the study area any person may be accused of witchcraft based on suspicion alone or general dislike and jealousy, anti-social behaviour, dreams, or divination. In such a situation people may change their behaviour in ways that minimize the chances of sparking off suspicion, to avoid being accused of witchcraft. For example, people may not give food gifts for fear of being accused of bewitching the food. Belief in witchcraft and its associated dangers have led people to devise ways to deal with it. A cleansing ritual (known as *kunyolewa* in Swahili) is one of the ways used to deal with witchcraft. Drawing on the literature (Green, 1993; 1994) and based on the information of key informants, who comprised people who participate in cleansing rituals and one person who worked as an assistant of cleansing specialists, the following section gives an account of the cleansing process. The cleansing ritual was once monopolized by the popular *Bibi* (grandmother) Kalembwani who was believed to have the power to deflate the influence of witches. It is said she got this power from her ancestors. She used to perform the cleansing ritual. After her death, her descendants took over. They have moved from Malinyi area in Ulanga District to Kiberege, Kilombero district. Many people from other regions in Southern Tanzania visit Kiberege for cleansing purposes.

People in Kilombero refer to this place as the 'salon' because the specialists use a combination of shaving and special medicines. The practices are supposed to suppress the powers of the witches and protect possible victims against bewitchment. For the Pogoro, the dominant ethnic group in Kilombero district, shaving is associated with cleansing and purification (Green, 1994). Many people in the village acknowledge that cleansing is done to restore peace and harmony in the community. Once purified, an individual will be regarded as a good person. Witchcraft accusations are difficult to prove. Someone can be accused of being a witch when caught red-handed by those who have special powers to identify witches, when they say ill words against others or are uncooperative. Accusations can also be due to improved wealth, which is always assumed to be at the expense of others, when one has a conflict with the accuser or when someone is always proud and boosting. Alternatively, people with problems like harvest failure, sickness and deaths may go to a witch doctor to find out who is causing troubles in their family. From there they get clues of who may be causing the problems; the witch doctor does not explicitly mention any name but only offers some hints.

Having identified a witch, the matter will be reported to the hamlet leader (previously chiefs) who summons the accused. While there, the accuser will touch the head of the accused with a coin, usually one hundred Tanzanian shillings. This act means that if the accused does not agree to be taken to the 'salon', the coins will be presented to the shaving specialist. They will work on the coin to make the accused go or deactivate his/her witchcraft power from a distance. Generally, though not always, the accuser and accused go together and sometimes the village authority provides them with someone to escort them, usually the village guard. The accuser has to pay for all travel expenses to go to the 'salon' and other costs involved including the fare for the guard (if provided). The accuser will have to bring a chicken and pay TShs. 2,020[4] for the cleansing rituals. Of this amount twenty shillings are for the ancestors (*mizimu*) and are kept in a special place. Both parties have to pay the costs of the return journey themselves.

Those who go the 'salon' (both accusers and accused) are supposed to spend the night there. They are not supposed to eat and to bath after midnight prior to the shaving day. On the shaving day all men and women have to go to the special shaving place dressed in their own old clothes, which will be discarded after the ritual. They are then shaved, men and women separately. The shaving is done by male assistants (*ndundame*) specialized in this job. The clients have to sit on a special seat sprinkled with medicine that supposedly causes discomfort to those who really practice witchcraft. A special instrument is used to shave all body hair, only for eye brows and armpit hair a razor blade is used. Women are asked to remove the hair from their private parts themselves. The old clothes worn during shaving have to be left at the 'salon' and those shaved put on new clothes. Specialists also apply special medicines on their heads, which should not be washed for a day.

After shaving the participants sit together at a specially medicated meal (*ugali*), which serves as a test: if there is a real witch among the group that person may not be able to direct food into her/his mouth but will smear it on her/his face and may do things which have been forbidden. Eating together is also a sign of a new beginning and that there is no threat from the accused anymore. It signifies reconciliation. Those involved are reconciled by shaking hands and warn the accused not to dare practicing or even to think about witchcraft again. Those who have shaved are given a certificate to prove to the community that they have been cleansed, implying that they cannot be accused as witches anymore because they lack the power to practice witchcraft again. People in the village say the process helps them to live in peace and solve witchcraft problems calmly, in contrast to what is happening in other parts of the country where the accused are killed, even if not confirmed to be witches. 'This is a peaceful way to resolve such problems', says one man. Villagers believe that shaving brings 'social health'. After shaving, witches cannot practice witchcraft and the possible victims are protected against bewitchment.

Sometimes force is used if the accused does not want to go to the 'salon' voluntarily. After the cleansing ritual it is assumed that the two parties involved will live on harmoniously, which is not always the case. Some people, especially newcomers in the area feel humiliated. Therefore, their relationship with the accuser will still be disturbed, although they keep up appearances. A woman who was once taken for cleansing said:

[4] One Euro was equivalent to an average of Tshs. 1,300 at the time of the study.

> *'Do you think I will relate well with such kind of person? We agree to go for shaving because people in this area regard it to be a way for reconciliation, so even we newcomers have to live like the natives otherwise you will not live peacefully. It is better to go to prove your innocence.'*

People I spoke to claimed to have been wrongly accused, but that they had to go to prove to the community that they are not witches because resistance may be interpreted as practicing witchcraft. Green (1994) found that in parts of Ulanga District, which shares more or less similar cultures with Kilombero district, some people choose to go for shaving on their own initiatives as a precaution against future witchcraft accusations. According to Green (2005) practices against witches contribute to the institutionalization of witchcraft in the area. Cleansing rituals are very common in the area; I came across many individuals who got involved in them. An individual may take two to three people for cleansing purposes. This has a very significant effect on household resources, which could have been used otherwise. Accusations of witchcraft are associated with decline in material and social well-being. Witchcraft cleansing causes significant losses in terms of time, money and other resources for households. Some people interviewed feel that cleansing rituals are an easy way of getting people's money, also because those who are conducting the rituals now are believed not to have the same powers as those in the past. Some people think that the practice results in hate instead of contributing to peace. In Mkamba witchcraft accusations seems to damage intra-community relations by eroding trust, which is the glue that holds communities together.

4.5.5 A livelihood profile

Farming employs a large percentage of village inhabitants. On average the size of the land owned between two to five acres. Some farmers have larger holdings and rent out to others. Access to land is very important for farming households. While by law women have the right to own land, in practice their ownership and control of land is not common (because of patrilineal inheritance). Where the household has land, it is usually owned and controlled by men and women have user rights only. Some women have land in their own right. They are mostly single, separated or divorced and have acquired the land by purchasing or have been given it by their family. When a man dies, the land is traditionally taken by his relatives and distributed among adult male children. Wives of the deceased are not entitled to land ownership under customary law. Cultural patterns of ownership, power and privilege limit the options available to some people while expanding those to others. Such norms are widespread in Tanzania and Mkamba village is not an exception. Many norms privilege men over women and adults over children. Currently some families resolve or mediate such issues in local courts where every immediate member of the family, including the wife, has an equal chance to inherit land and other properties.

Most of the Mkamba people do not have farming plots near the village; they farm in distant farms plots. Since most households farm away from the village, they are forced to stay on the farms during the farming season, usually from December to August (Figure 4.2). It is not possible to commute because of the long distances and lack of income for daily fares. In case of a short distance, bicycles are used to go to the fields and for transport of farm harvests. The traditional crops produced in distant farms are rice and maize, mostly mono-cropped. These crops are rain-fed,

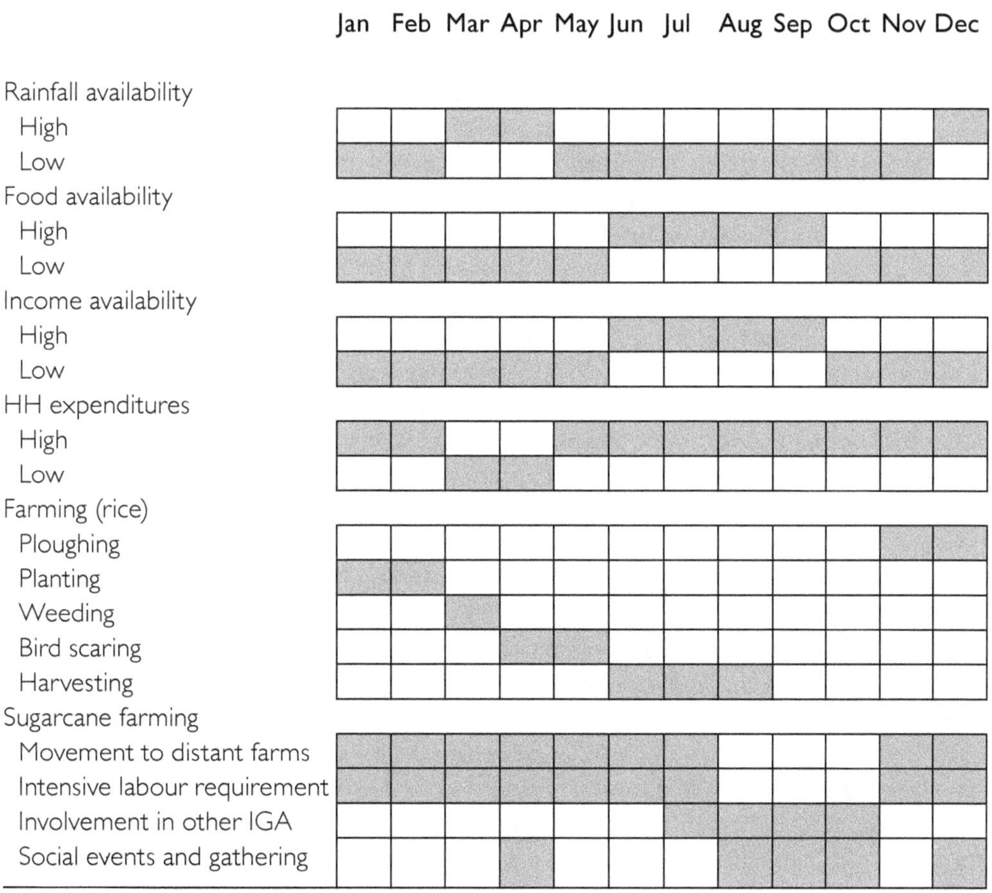

Source: Focus Group Discussion no 5 (See Table 3.2).

Figure 4.2. Seasonal calendar of Mkamba village.

no irrigation is practiced. Most cultivation is done manually by hand hoe, using one's own family labour. Some households hire tractors for ploughing, the other operations being done by members of the household unless they can afford to hire people. Hiring extra labour is often difficult because of cash shortages during crucial farming periods, and because labour may be in short supply when people are busy on their own farms. In distant farms some poor farmers sell their labour to get cash to invest in their own farms, which reduces the time for working on their own plots. Although for many farmers in the area food self-sufficiency seems to be a priority, nearly all of them are involved in marketing. They either sell or buy cash crops (mainly rice and maize) locally or to/from outside the village. However, returns from agriculture are low. Structural adjustment policies have also contributed to the failure of smallholder farmers to sustain farm production and provide for their families (Kashuliza & Mbiha, 1995).

People spend more time on farming than on other income-generating activities. There are numerous expenditures after harvest. Money or food is needed for different purposes such as group contributions, ceremonies, and village contributions for school and hospital construction and other public facilities. It is apparent that most of the household's cash or food supplies are exhausted before the next farming season, forcing many to seek loans to invest in farming. Usually people get loans from moneylenders in the village, which are repaid in kind after harvest. According to the Village Report (2003) only 65 percent of the population has sufficient food throughout the year or has a seasonal shortage, 35 percent is chronically food insecure. Many times, poor farmers are so short of money that they are forced to sell a substantial proportion of crops soon after harvest, when prices are often low. They then have to buy food or seed at much higher prices later in the season, which paves the way for a vicious cycle of food insecurity.

Though farming employs the majority of the village population, because of its precarious nature, many people have diversified their livelihood portfolios. Farming no longer enjoys the monopoly it once had. In the study area declining farm incomes, increased pressure on land, and opportunities created by economic liberalization have given rise to a dynamic rural informal sector. Mkamba villagers have diversified their livelihood portfolios to include off-farm and non-farm activities. Trading and services provision have become prominent activities in the village. They include food vending, local brewing, operating market stalls and kiosks, livestock keeping, running milling machines, renting houses, gardening, crop marketing and providing services such as tailoring, hair dressing, masonry, carpentry and traditional treatment. It helps that Mkamba is easy accessible, which facilitates transportation of goods to and from the area. A wide range of natural resources are also tapped. However, because there is a very strict control on the use of forest resources by the Udzungwa

Mountains National Park, villagers who used to collect firewood from the forest are only allowed to do this for two days a week (Fridays and Sundays). Becausc of this, most of them are obliged to use charcoal. Hence, charcoal-selling has become an important source of income for some households, as is brick-production. Some of the villagers are employed in the sugar factory, the hydro-electric power station and other institutions in the village such as banks, schools, the dispensary, and village/ward offices. Though employed, they still do farming.

Some people in the study area sell their labour as a livelihood strategy and as a way of coping with problems. Most of them are hired to work on paddy and sugar plots. They are enumerated according to the *mraba* system, in which a paddy plot sized 10 x 10 steps yields wages of TShs. 2,000. The daily wages for working on sugar cane plots depend on the agreement with the plot owner. If one is hired to work on the Company's plantations, the daily wages are TShs. 1,800. Gender differentiation is visible in the type of informal sector employment, with women more involved in typical female activities, such as beer brewing, food preparation and sale, and sewing.

Migration of people to Mkamba village because of the employment opportunities offered by the sugar cane estates and the growing cash economy and trade opportunities resulted in increased population pressure on the land. Not only does migration cause land shortage, but it also increases cultural diversity, which may affect the social cohesion in the community. In the case of communities living in the eastern part of the Udzungwa Mountains National Park cultural diversity has influenced the implementation of environmental conservation and other development programs (Kikula *et al.*, 2003). At the same time, many of the migrants who decided to settle in the village ended up losing their links with their place of origin. They can neither rely on their kin anymore for assistance when needed nor be relied upon to give assistance to their relatives in their area of origin.

4.5.6 History and significance of the sugar plantation in the area

The Kilombero sugar cane estate occupies 8,000 hectares of land. The survey and initial soil tests were done in 1957 by experts from the Netherlands. The factory was constructed and started operating in 1960 as a parastatal company under the Sugar Development Corporation (SUDECO). Sugar production showed declining trends in the mid-1980's due to climatic and socio-economic problems. When the sugar estate was established, the government sought to increase out-growers' production to offer rural self-employment to the people surrounding the estate. Theoretically, the estate was to provide support to out-growers such as credits, machinery for land preparation, and assistance with harvesting and transporting cane. However, the state management experienced high costs, hence scaled down its support to out-growers. There was a decline in managerial efficiency, profitability and investment levels. As a result, the annual production declined and the sugarcane factory was under-utilized. During the mid-1990s annual production started to increase, mainly in response to favourable economic situation in the country following trade liberalization. The public sugar company was sold under the on-going privatization schemes in Tanzania and since 1997 is owned by ILLOVO Sugar Company of Natal, South Africa. The company owns the land through a 99-years lease. It owns two large scale plantations, Kilombero One (K1) and Kilombero Two (K2), which are the major sources of raw materials for its factory.

Before the privatization of the sugar company in 1998, many Kilombero sugar cane out-growers lacked the necessary capital, technology, and training to take advantage of the improving market. Low capitalization hindered rehabilitation of older farms and the purchase of tools, fertilizers, and high-quality cane seed. Inadequate loading services prevented farmers from harvesting and delivering their cane when sugar content peaks. Poor cane-husbandry methods significantly reduced average yields per hectare. These problems have been largely solved since the Kilombero Sugar Company purchased the state-owned sugar processing plant and made considerable investments in its rehabilitation. The company's rapid expansion has boosted local demand for raw sugar cane and provided thousands of independent cane growers with new opportunities to expand their production, sales and personal incomes. Sugar cane production by out-growers has increased significantly from 68,000 tons in 2001 to 240,000 tons in 2004. The company strengthened the out-growers cane association (KCGA) that is responsible for coordinating all the activities pertaining to sugar cane production and sales as well as defending farmers' interests. The association was established in 1991 with 350 members and now counts about 2,500 members from various villages in Kilombero district. The company offers extension services and other services such as cane cutting, loading and transport of cane from the field to the factory. The costs related to these services are later deducted from the payments to the farmers. The company has also created and contracted sustainable businesses to other stakeholders. These include loading and hauling activities, input supplies and technical support and services. The existence of the company in the area has stimulated the economy of the area by creating a ready market for food crops and other items from the adjacent small-scale producers. The company provides basic social services to the community surrounding it. It has the hospital, primary and secondary schools offering services also to other members of the community. On the whole the existence of the company in the area has increased the choices available to the population of Mkamba. However, privatization has not been without costs to the Mkamba community.

Effects of privatization

As was reported in the Focus Groups 1 and 2 (see Table 3.2) the privatization of the sugarcane estate has entailed the following negative consequences for the Mkamba people:

- *Split households and double homesteads*: Those who used to farm nearby the village were compelled to move and work in distant farms for longer periods. During the farming period parents and other adults in households move to the farms, leaving behind school-age children and young ones. Consequently those left behind get no proper care. They are left with very few resources to live on, leading some of them to seeking alternative ways of survival such as engaging in transactional sex (by girls) and theft (by boys). Such strategies expose girls to the risks of pregnancy and HIV infection. School absenteeism is also high during this period. Generally, conditions in the distant farms are very poor, there is no clean water and there are plenty of mosquitoes, increasing the likelihood of contracting waterborne diseases and malaria. In some places there are no roads and if there are they become impassable during the rainy season, which makes transport of inputs difficult. The company draws labour from other regions in the country, mostly Mbeya and Iringa during the peak season (June- December. As men migrate to work in the sugarcane plantations women are left behind to care for the household. Some of the labourers eventually decide to settle in the village at the end of their seasonal contracts.
- *Disruption of small-scale farming*: Before the privatization of the sugar company, many Mkamba households were producing food crops on unused company plots. Though legally the land belonged to the sugar company, the law was not enforced and the local people could use the land. After privatization, all plots were reclaimed and villagers were barred from these plots. Those who legally owned plots near the sugarcane plantation could no longer produce other crops than sugarcane because they would not flourish near sugarcane and because of crop predators such as monkeys and vermin hiding in the sugarcane farms around. So, production of other crops like rice, maize and vegetables became difficult; forcing people to produce food on distant farms. All this had a big impact on household food security in the area. Many people were forced to look for new land in other villages. Some cleared bushes and forests in distant villages to get arable land. Those who were not able to get virgin land, hired land on a short-term basis at prices between TShs. 15,000 and to 25,000 per acre per farming season.
- *Market monopoly*: Despite the fact that the Company offers a reliable market, it does not buy more sugarcane from out-growers once it has reached its production targets. Farmers whose sugarcane is not purchased suffer significant loss.

Furthermore, the retrenchment policy of the company caused many people to become unemployed and face difficulties in re-establishing their livelihoods. Some of them are desperate and live in destitute conditions. Additionally, the company is criticized for the low wages it pays to its employees.

Sugarcane out-growers scheme

Sugarcane out-growers supply the bulk of the cane for the factory. Most out-growers grow the cane in small farms with sizes ranging from 1 to 5 acres, and only a small number of farmers have plots more than ten acres. Out-growers sugarcane is grown as a dry-land crop and is rain-fed. Most people produce cane on their own plots, others farm on hired plots. Villagers who have plots near the village and cannot invest in sugarcane farming, sell or hire-out their plots to those who are able to grow sugarcane. Renting-out one acre costs TShs. 100,000 to 150,000 per year. It is usually done for a minimum of five years. Sugarcane out-growers from 32 groups in Kilombero district produce cane from about 5,203 ha (equivalent to 13,007 acres). The figures in Table 4.3 indicate the increased area cultivated by out-growers, their share increasing from 35 percent in 1997/98 to 57 percent in 2003/04.

Any villager can become a sugarcane out-grower provided s/he has resources to invest in cane farming. Still each out-grower must be a member of a village producer group to be able to benefit from and get access the services offered by

Table 4.3. Sugar production 1997/98 to 2003/04 of Kilombero Sugar Company.

Year	Area covered	Sugar cane harvested (tons)	Sugar produced (tons)	Sugar cane area coverage in hactares (%)	
				Sugar plantation plots	Out growers plots
1997/98	7,917.5	387,820.5	29,517.0	43.2	35.0
1998/99	8,886.4	454,787.3	42,062.0	42.9	35.0
1999/00	9,262.8	533,492.3	50,159.0	64.0	43.0
2000/01	9,347.7	544,792.0	61,890.0	73.2	37.0
2001/02	10,079.2	641,679.0	72,498.7	75.1	45.4
2002/03	12,539.8	849,350.0	98,412.6	77.8	48.7
2003/04	13,784.0	1,095,126.0	126,743.0	86.1	57.0

Source: Kilombero District Report, 2004.

the out-grower cane association (KCGA) and the Sugar Company. The members have to pay an entrance fee (of about TShs. 3,000) and make annual contributions. Upon registration members are given an identification number that is used in all transactions with the company. All village producer groups are represented in the KCGA. The organizational structure of KCGA is shown in Figure 4.3.

Leaders of village out-growers groups represent their members to the KCGA. This is the body responsible for linking sugar cane out-growers with the company. The KCGA is responsible for defending farmers' interests by negotiating with the company management on issues related to pricing, cane supply to the factory and availability of farm implements. The KCGA also offers training to its members on proper sugar cane husbandry. The company has facilitated and strengthened the association by offering technical back-up and linking it with various financial institutions.

Since sugarcane production requires heavy investment in terms of inputs, most growers get loans to invest in their plots. It is only through the sugarcane out-growers village groups and the KCGA, that an individual loan application to the local Saving-and-Credit Cooperatives (SACCOs) can be processed. Groups present the total loan request of their members to the KCGA which then submits it to the SACCOS. The village group acts as a guarantor for its members requesting loans. To be eligible for a loan one has to be a member of the saving-and-credit association. To become a member one has to pay an entry fee of TShs. 5,000 and have a minimum of ten shares worth TShs. 10,000 each.

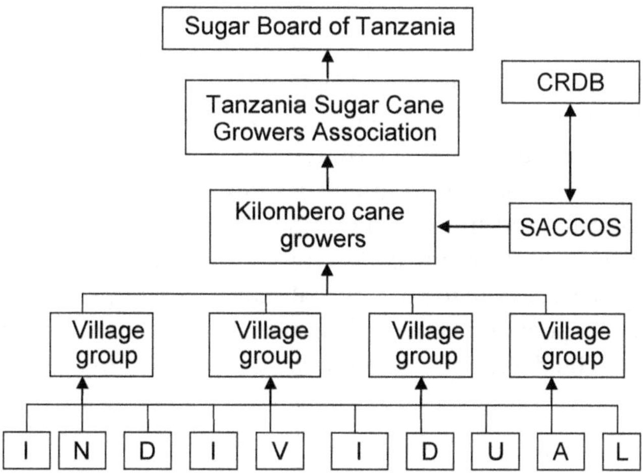

Figure 4.3. Organizational structure of sugar cane out-growers in Kilombero.

A loan applicant has to attach payment slips from the Sugar Company showing the total income from his/her previous sales to the factory. This condition is difficult to meet for people who have never previously engaged in sugarcane farming. Basically sugarcane production is only possible for well-to-do farmers who can get the initial capital to invest in sugarcane farming and can afford the payments. Even though sugarcane out-growers are encouraged to take loans from the local saving-and credit association, some get loans from other sources like the National Microfinance Bank (NMB) and from moneylenders in the village.

4.5.7 Wealth profile of households in the village

To capture the qualitative aspects of socio-economic well-being, the villagers' own perceptions of poverty and wealthy were explored as well. During the discussion in Focus Group 5 it was found that poverty is thought to be the result of many, often mutually reinforcing, factors, including lack of productive resources to generate material wealth as well as non-material well-being such as education and good health. During the focus group discussion it appeared that for the participants household wealth is not only associated with material well-being only but also intangible aspects. They emphasized that household wealth has to do with the ability to provide for its members and pay for school fees and medical expenses. Table 4.4 outlines the criteria and attributes which Mkamba villagers use to determine the wealth of households.

4.6 Concluding notes

This chapter has given a descriptive account of the changing economic and social environment in which the Mkamba people are living. Many households in the study area are vulnerable and insecure, due to lack of land and other resources, chronic and prolonged illness, witchcraft accusations, and low incomes because of distant farming and falling agricultural productivity. Though offering new opportunities, privatization has also contributed to impoverishing the community. The village is affected by overlapping and interacting vulnerabilities, including the HIV/AIDS pandemic, which threatens the entire community. Against this background, important questions emerge. These pertain to how mutual sharing and support has been affected by HIV/AIDS and how poor and vulnerable households cope in the changing context. These questions will be dealt with in following chapters of this publication.

Table 4.4. Profile of households in Mkamba village according to wealth.

Criteria	Rich household	Moderately poor household	Poor household
Housing	Owns huge permanent houses with iron roof, electricity and water. Owns houses for rent and wholesale shop.	Owns a good house made of bricks and iron roofing with water, electricity and other facilities.	Either owns mud bricks and grass-roofed house or relies on renting poor quality rooms, and sometimes unable to pay rent.
Land	Owns large plots of land; uses tractors and hires people to work on the farm.	Owns farms plots from 5 acres and above, use tractors and can hire extra labour.	Small plots below 5 acres. Hires farming plots after selling their own plots and uses hand hoe.
Selling labour	Does not sell labour.	Does not sell labour.	Sells labour for more than three months.
Assets	Owns cars, tractors milling machines, mobile phone and wholesale shops.	Owns motorcycle/ bicycles, mobile phone and a medium retail shop.	Few household assets and furniture.
Loans availability	Get loàns easily because having collateral.	Gets loans easier from institutions because having assets as collateral.	Dependent on moneylenders for loans at high interest rates.
Food security status	Has no food shortages and has enough or more food reserve for the whole year.	Has seasonal food shortages but can cope, food stocks last for about 3-6 months.	Chronic food shortages with food stocks lasting for less than 3 months, adopting dangerous coping responses like selling sex and, stealing
Number of children	Small number of children.	Average number of children.	Large family with many dependants.
Number of friends	Many friends.	Good number of friends.	Few friends.
Membership in groups	Member of groups.	Member of groups.	Not member of groups.
Participation in communal work	Gives money instead of participating in communal activities.	Participates or give money.	Usually participates in communal activities with own-labour.

Table 4.4. Continued.

Criteria	Rich household	Moderately poor household	Poor household
Education	Can educate all their children.	Possibility of educating 1or 2 children.	Children are not educated, do casual labour like brick-making, paddy-drying, and domestic work.
Children's condition	Children are cheerful and well dressed.	Children are cheerful and well dressed.	Children are poorly dressed and timid. Girls get pregnant; many boys are thieves and pickpockets. Problems of drug addiction.
Mobility	Very mobile.	Mobile.	Mobility is restricted.
Meeting household needs	Are able to meet household needs	Are able to meet household needs.	Unable to meet family basic needs – food, clothes, health, education
Medical care	Gets treatment from traditional healers for other reasons but not lack of money.	Gets treatment from traditional healers for other reasons but not lack of money.	Goes to traditional healers for treatment because cannot afford the expenses of public or private hospitals/ clinics.

Source: Focus Group 5 (see Table 3.2).

Chapter 5
Economic and social impacts of HIV/AIDS at the household level

As discussed in Chapter 2, it is important to study HIV/AIDS impacts on social capital in relation to other resources. This chapter aims at providing an understanding of the impacts of HIV/AIDS on the different sets of assets that are essential to households' livelihoods. The chapter shows that for many households the burden of ill-health, caring for the chronically ill, premature death and caring for AIDS orphans is manifested through the depletion of human, financial and physical assets, and the disruption of social support mechanisms. HIV/AIDS exacerbates existing rural problems such as food insecurity and poverty. It has a greater impact on poor than better-off households as it forces the former to draw on their already limited resources in order to cushion the shock. This threatens their ability to respond to future insecurity. Gender and age are important attributes that determine HIV/AIDS impacts. Although HIV/AIDS impacts resemble other shocks, they differ in the way they affect the labour potential of adults in their prime years and in the way in which the impacts are gendered. The results presented in this chapter are generated from case studies, focused group discussions and the household survey.

5.1 Characteristics of the respondents

It is important to describe the characteristic of the respondents because they have a bearing on other issues investigated in the study. A total of 180 respondents were interviewed in the survey of which 55 percent were men and 45 percent were women.

Most of respondents (77%) were 15 to 59 years old, 23 percent were aged above 59. A high percentage of respondents were in their productive and reproductive prime age. Most of the respondents were married, as shown in Table 5.1. However, more than half of the female respondents were not currently married at the time of survey, while most of male respondents were. This can be explained by the fact that men who are divorced or widowed can easily remarry. Male-headed household accounted for 79 percent of the households and 19.5 (n = 35) percent were female-headed households and 1.5 (n = 2) percent were child-headed households.

The average household size in the sample is 5.1, which is slightly higher than the national average of 4.9 (URT, 2003a). Household headship is associated with

Table 5.1. Marital status by sex of the respondents (N=180).

	Sex of respondent			
	Women		Men	
	Frequency	Percent	Frequency	Percent
Married	37	45.7	86	86.9
Single	16	19.7	2	2.0
Widowed	11	13.6	3	3.0
Divorced/separated	17	21.0	8	8.1
Total	81	100	99	100

Source: Household survey, 2005.

household size ($\chi^2 = 10.221$, $p = 0.017$). Female-headed households are smaller than male-headed ones.

Of the household members in the sample 426 (47.2%) were men, while 477 (52.7%) were women. The sex-age structure of household membership is shown in Figure 5.1. The narrowing base in the age-groups of 0-4 and 5-9 suggests a decline in fertility or an increase in child mortality. The few men and women in the 40-59 age-brackets may indicate young adult mortality, probably due to AIDS. Additionally, there are always sex-ratio imbalances in an area with a lot of migration.

Table 5.2. Household size (N=180).

Number of household members	Frequency	Percent
1	10	5.6
2-4	69	38.3
5-8	87	48.3
9 and above	14	7.8
Total	180	100

Source: Household survey, 2005.

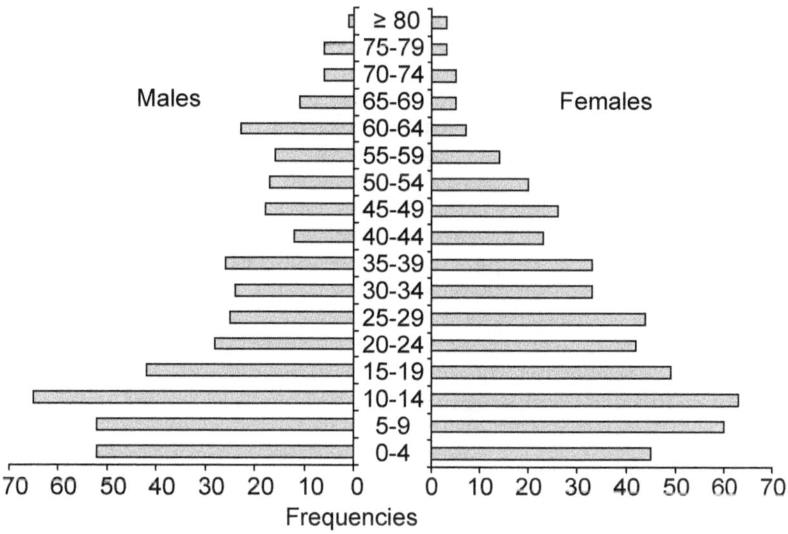

Figure 5.1. Respondent's age-sex structure (N=903).

Most of the respondents (81%) have attained primary education. These high percentages are the result of universal and compulsory primary education in Tanzania and adult education campaigns in the country. Of the respondents six percent have secondary and college education and 13 percent had no formal education.

Table 5.3 presents the distribution of household types. It shows that 46.7 percent of the households interviewed are extended-family based and 45.5 percent consists of nuclear-family based households. The relatively high percentage of the latter type may be related to in-migration (see also Tables 5.4 and 5.5). Some of the

Table 5.3. Type of household (N=180).

Type of household	Frequency	Percent
Extended family household	83	46.2
Nuclear family household	82	45.5
Household with non-family members	5	2.7
One person household	10	5.6
Total	180	100.0

Source: Household survey, 2005.

migrant households have lost all contact with relatives in their place of origin. Though household membership is primarily based on marital and kinship ties, some households have members who are not biologically related. Households with non-family members (2.8%) are those that employ people to help in household and farming activities. Only a small proportion of the respondents are in polygamous marriages, which is due to the fact that most of respondents are Christians (45.6% and 17.7% Roman Catholic and Protestant respectively) who are not allowed to have more than one partner. About 36 percent of the respondents are Muslims.

The majority of the respondents have lived in the village for more than ten years (Table 5.4), but only ten percent of the respondents were born there. This suggests that most of them moved in from different parts of the country for employment and business purposes.

Place of origin of the respondents is shown in Table 5.5. More than half of those interviewed came from within Morogoro Region (51%). The second region of origin is Mbeya, followed by Iringa. People from Mbeya and Iringa are mostly found in the area during the sugar-cane harvesting period when seasonal labour is recruited from these regions, and some of them decided to settle in the village. There are also people from other regions who are working or have previously worked with the Sugar Company and who have decided to settle in the village after retrenchment.

Rural households in Tanzania have many and varied sources of income as compared to households in urban areas (URT, 2002). Farming was reported to be the main livelihood activity by 80.6 percent of the respondents. About 16 percent are involved in non-farm activities such as livestock-keeping, trade and artisan work as major livelihood activities and only 3.3 percent are employed. Although farming is still a major occupation, there are no households that can live from farming only. People engage in non-farm activities to supplement their income. Remittances have been

Table 5.4. Duration of stay in the village (N=180).

Duration (years)	Frequency	Percent
Since birth	18	10.0
Below 10 years	27	15.0
More than 10 years	135	75.0
Total	180	100.0

Source: Household survey, 2005.

Table 5.5. Region of origin of household head.

Region	Frequency	Percent
Morogoro	92	51.1
Iringa	17	9.5
Ruvuma	15	8.3
Mbeya	24	13.3
Kilimanjaro	4	2.2
Coastal region	4	2.2
Mwanza/Shinyanga	7	3.9
Dodoma	7	3.9
Others[1]	10	5.6
Total	180	100

[1] Respondents from Tanga (2), Mara (2), Bukoba (2), Lindi (2), Kigoma (3) and Kenya (1).
Source: Household survey, 2005.

appreciated as another source of income. About 43 percent of respondents admitted to having been sent cash, food, clothes or other items by household members residing elsewhere, but did not specify how often. By diversifying income sources households may reduce risks and increase livelihood security.

5.2 The impact of HIV/AIDS on household assets and livelihood activities

HIV/AIDS impacts have brought about a wide range of changes in people's livelihood assets and activities. As we will see in the following sections, HIV/AIDS strips individuals and households assets and resources that are important for their livelihood.

5.2.1 Effects on human capital

The most direct impact of HIV/AIDS on households relates to the loss of human capital that enables people to work and use their skills and knowledge, which is crucial in pursuing livelihood activities. HIV/AIDS impacts on human capital are caused by morbidity and mortality of household members. About 29 percent (n = 53) of the households interviewed had experienced deaths of one or more household members. Causes of the death are shown in Table 5.6.

Table 5.6. Self-reported cause of death of household members (N=53).

Cause of death	Frequency	Percent
Respiratory problems[1]	14	21.2
Cardiovascular problems[2]	10	15.2
Stomach pains	9	13.6
AIDS	6	9.1
Malaria	18	27.3
Others[3]	9	13.6
Total	66	100

[1] Pneumonia, TB, and other respiratory problems.
[2] Heart and blood pressure related problems.
[3] Appendix, liver, kidneys, mental problems, accidents and old age.
Source: Household survey, 2005.

Though only 9.1 percent deaths were said to be caused by AIDS, one may suspect that many deaths are caused by AIDS-related infections, such as pneumonia and TB. It has to be noted that the true burden of AIDS mortality might be hidden in reported causes of death. Respondents were more open about someone in the household having died of AIDS than about someone being sick, for fear of stigmatization or rejection.

Table 5.7 shows that about 65 percent of all deaths were of individuals at prime productive age, namely between the ages of 15 and 64. Most of those died were adult sons or daughters of the household head. Women accounted for a slightly higher percentage of the deaths that occurred during ten years prior to the survey than men. These results highlight the effect of the epidemic on the current and future supply of labour and the likely implications for household earning capacities. Both domestic labour and productive activities are at stake when women die. Although in many instances medical evidence on the cause of death of individuals was not available and most of the respondents were not open about the cause of death of deceased household members, from the age distribution it seems reasonable to infer that AIDS accounts for a large proportion of deaths.

Changes in household composition as a result of household members moving in and out are another notable effect brought about by HIV/AIDS. Affected households may react to HIV/AIDS impacts by either bringing in new people or sending away others. In this study, changes in household composition were elicited by questioning the

Table 5.7. Reported deaths in the sample households by age and sex of the deceased during ten years prior to the survey (N=66).

Age group of the deceased	Women		Men		Total	
	(N)	Percent	(N)	Percent	(N)	Percent
< 15	7	23.3	3	8.3	10	15.1
15-64	21	70.0	22	61.1	43	65.2
≥ 64	2	6.7	11	30.6	13	19.7
Total	30	100	36	100	66	100

Source: Household survey, 2005.

respondents about the number of individuals who moved into or out of the household during the past ten years. Forty-one households (22.8 %) received people who were previously not members of the household. In two cases the persons who moved in previously had their own household which had ceased to exist. Dissolution of households is a much observed phenomenon in high-prevalence areas (Rugalema, 1999; Barnett & Whiteside, 2002). Seven out of forty-one households received more than one person during the recall period. Table 5.8 shows that a considerable proportion (44.3%) were dependants (elderly and young). The reasons for moving in varied. Children moved in to get help in providing for their basic needs including education, adults moved in for reasons of care, work or marriage. Out of 30 HIV/AIDS-affected households identified in the study five households received young adults who were ill who moved in for care.

Table 5.8. Persons moving in during the ten years prior to the survey by age and sex (N=41).

Age group of the person	Women		Men		Total	
	(N)	Percent	(N)	Percent	(N)	Percent
< 15	12	37.5	9	45.0	21	40.4
15 - 64	18	56.3	11	55.0	29	55.7
≥ 65	2	6.2	0	0.0	2	3.9
Total	32	100	20	100	52	100

Source: Household survey 2005.

Household member out-migration is another effect of the AIDS pandemic. When parents die, children go to live with other relatives or care for themselves. In the sample there were only two HIV/AIDS-affected households that sent away children to another household. However, because many households do not have strong ties with the members of their kinship network, sending the children or other dependants to relatives is often not an option. I came across dependants such as elderly, children and physically unfit people who could not get family support and were destitute and living in misery. As for children who are orphans, they are too young to leave the village, so they remain in the village and live on charity, which is not easily available, or work as casual labourers or domestic helpers.

The impact of HIV/AIDS on household labour availability is not only direct but also indirect, because productive time is diverted to taking care of the sick. HIV/AIDS-affected individuals incur productivity losses as a result of their illness. Illness of household members decreases the number of household members who are able to participate full-time in domestic and productive activities. In Mkamba, households that take care of people suffering from with AIDS or other chronic diseases, whether or not AIDS-related, face severe labour constraints. In total, 45 households had 53 ill young adults who were unable to work. Out of 30 HIV/AIDS-affected households identified, 15 households had people who had been sick for more than six months. Depending on their composition such households are likely to have a high 'effective dependency ratio'. De Waal & Whiteside (2003) defined the term effective dependency ratio to include normal demographic dependants as well as adults aged between 18 and 59 who are unable to work. Dependants who are coming back home because they are terminally ill and need care and orphans who join the household result in an increasing dependency ratio (Table 5.9), although

Table 5.9. Effective dependency ratio for HIV/AIDS-affected and unaffected households in percentages (N=180).

Household HIV/ AIDS status	Effective dependency ratio			Total
	Low (0.0-0.33)	Medium (0.34-0.66)	High (> 0.66)	
Affected	16.7	43.3	40.0	16.7
Non-affected	34.0	34.0	32.0	83.3
Total	31.1	35.6	33.3	100

$\chi2$= 3.50, p=0.173.
Source: Household survey, 2005.

it is not statistically significant. This causes the effective dependency ratio in HIV/AIDS-affected households to be slightly higher than that in non-affected households, implying that the former have a smaller supply of labour than the latter.

Table 5.10 shows no significant association between household headship and dependency ratio, even though female-headed households have higher effective dependency ratios than their male counterparts. The smaller household size (see above) and higher dependency ratio (though not significant) of female-headed households mean that they are likely to experience more labour shortages than male-headed households.

Table 5.10. Effective dependency ratio by household headship in percentages (N=180).

Household headship	Effective dependency ratio			Total
	Low (0.0-0.33)	Medium (0.34-0.66)	High (>0.66)	
Male	34.3	35.0	30.7	79.4
Female	18.9	37.8	43.2	20.6
Total	31.1	35.6	33.3	100

$\chi 2$= 3.66, p=0.160.
Source: Household survey, 2005.

Effects on children

The HIV/AIDS pandemic has resulted in an increase of orphans and in problems in meeting the necessary needs of orphaned children. Children are living with and caring for sick and dying parents, or living in a household that has taken in orphans. Cases 5.1 and 5.2 illustrate how orphans cope with the impact of their parents' illness and death and how they are adjusting to the new reality.

The two cases depict that in the absence of other healthy persons to look after the sick, children are responsible for the care and support of their sick parents. At times such children cannot get food, they wander in the community hoping for someone to sympathize with their situation and give them food. They are forced to work to boost household earnings in order to buy food. In addition, their education suffers because of missed school days or drop out because school fees and other necessary

Case 5.1. Naomi: double orphan, loss of skills, change in livelihood activities.

Naomi is 16 years old and has completed primary school in 2003. Her parents, who were farmers, have died. The father (38) died in 1995 and the mother (35) in 2005. After her father's death, Naomi's mother moved to her par-ents' house with the children. Naomi's mother was not recognized as a legal wife by her husband's relatives because of religious differences. Since Naomi's mother was a Roman Catholic and the man was a Muslim, they did not have their marriage registered. While in her parents' home, Naomi's mother worked in the dried fish business, travelling between Ifakara and Mkamba. She had another baby from another man but the baby died at the age of two. After her child's death, she started experiencing recurrent illnesses until she died in 2005. She sold a radio to meet her medical ex-penses. Naomi said her mother was diagnosed with typhoid.

Naomi and her two brothers stayed with their sick mother at her grandparents' house but life was very difficult, since the elderly couple could not properly look after them. Naomi got pregnant and had a baby who was ten months old at the time of this interview. After her mother's burial, Naomi was taken to her in-laws' house although Naomi's partner was not living there. He went to Dar es Salaam after Naomi got pregnant but came back with mental problems for which he was treated by a traditional healer. The couple shares meals with Naomi's in-laws and have been given one room in the compound. She has to go to the field with her in-laws, work that she finds difficult. She had never done farming work when her parents were alive. She says that farming is very hard but that she has no other options. She has to do the work with the baby on her back and, when she returns home has to make food for the family. She can-not earn money, for example by making rice buns, because she lacks capital and skills. She has no one to turn to for assistance. She knows how to make bread, since she used to see her mother doing it. She liked to learn tailoring but her mum who would have paid for her fees fell sick and later died.

Her mother left few assets like furniture and kitchen items, which will be distributed to children and relatives on the day marking the end of the mourning period. The ceremony for the end of the mourning period should have been held long ago, but Naomi's grandparents and other relatives have no money to organize it. Since her mother had one acre of rice land, she expects that the harvest from it will be used to perform this ceremony.

contributions cannot be paid. As with Naomi (Case 5.1), girls are forced to get married at early age to cope with the absence of their parents. Due to the economic pressure experienced by Naomi's grandparents, they could not to abide by any marriage norms; the girl was just handed over to the in-laws. This indicates that HIV/AIDS impacts also changes the norms which people used to observe.

Case 5.2. Castor: paternal orphan, children-headed household.

Castor is 11 years old and is in class four in one of the village schools. He is living with his brother, who is 14. Two of his sisters got married, one in the village and the other in another village. Their mother divorced and re-married another man in the village. After their mother's divorce in 2002, their father became sick and died in 2005 after a prolonged illness. Castor and his brother were the ones who looked after him. They had to cook, wash clothes and get some medi-cation for him. Sometimes their mother would visit them and help them with domestic chores. When his father was hospitalized Castor's sister used to make food and visit him in the hospital.
Castor and his brother manage their own household. The brother works to get money and cooks while Castor washes the dishes and cleans the house. They get some money from the big cooking pan they rented to the pork butchery, where it is used for making soup. They are paid TShs. 300 everyday and they use the money to buy half a kilogram of rice and beans for a day. In most cases, they don't eat during the day time but only at night. When they don't have food, Castor sometimes goes to his mother for food or money. There are times she has nothing to give, so he goes to school without eating or does not go at all. His brother does not like going to their mother's new family. Occasionally their sister, who married in the village, gives them some cash, but this is never enough. His brother looks for casual jobs to get money for food. Castor said that when their father was well they had three meals a day, but now they usually only have one meal. When their father died he left them with a four-room house, furniture and kitchen items. They also have a farm which is rented. The money was taken by their cousin, who was supposed to give them money for daily expenses but is not doing so.

To cope with their parents' deaths, as it is with Naomi (Case 5.1) girls may seek adult protection by getting married early to seek economic security. Removal of children from school due to lack of income has a long-term effect on human capital. Girls are particularly disadvantaged because for them education is a tool of empowerment, important for changing women's subordinate status in society. Educated girls and women can venture into businesses to earn an income for themselves and their families, which would make them less vulnerable to HIV-infection. Since most of the HIV/AIDS-affected households in the area are poor with very few options left to mitigate AIDS-impacts, they may respond in ways that expose them to irreversible long-term effects. Children are forced into adult roles immaturely. They have to work to provide for themselves and their siblings. Child-headed households tend to be among the poorest, with older siblings often having to work in order to take care of the younger ones. In some cases, like that of Castor (Case 5.2), relatives who ought to be caretakers, seize the few resources that the orphans could use such as land, household furniture and bicycles. When too young and inexperienced to manage the land inherited they could be provided with money from the rented plot to cover for their expenses. However, as in Castor's case, children may be too young to claim their rights and the caretaker may take advantage of their vulnerable position.

Traditionally, there are informal arrangements to take care of bereaved children. In many cases grandparents take over. However, the costs to provide for additional children discourage family members to take them in, as shown in the case of Naomi. Lack of basic resources, such as food and money may partly contribute to the refusal of kin to support the orphans. In some cases orphaned children are not cared for at all, forcing children to assume household headship.

Effects on elderly

Normal life cycle patterns are reversed with HIV/AIDS. Children die before their parents, leaving grandparents to look after themselves at a time when they might have looked forward to get support from their children. Grandparents have to assume responsibilities of a parent once again and care for grandchildren orphaned by the loss of their own parents. The following case shows the many difficulties elderly households face and how they are trying to manage the situation.

Case 5.3 describes the circumstances commonly found in households that have experienced young-adult deaths. Elderly women and men are needed to support grandchildren and other sick members of the family. Out of 30 HIV/AIDS-affected households, seven households received young adults who came to their parents for care. Sick young adults come home for care when normally they would have their own household away from home and supported their elderly parents. The care-giving burden falls disproportionately on women, especially mothers. Men also help, but their role is more limited: they are expected to provide financial resources, in which they not always succeed. During the Focus Group Discussion (FGD 8, see Table 3.2) it transpired that apart from providing financial resources, men may also be involved in giving practical care if the sick person is a man. Most of the elderly-headed households depend on their children's support, which means their death makes them economically and socially weak and in addition they have to foster the orphans left by their children.

Elderly women in particular face enormous responsibilities without having the financial and other resources they need. They have to care for their sick children and orphaned grandchildren, without having adequate economic, social and physical resources. They usually also lack the support of extended family members or other social support systems. In this situation elderly women are forced to undertake

Case 5.3. Mama Mkago: looking after grandchildren.

Mama Mkago is in her early sixties living with her last-born daughter and three orphans from her four daughters who died in 1998, 1999, 2000 and 2005. The last daughter died when this study was conducted, and four months later the baby she left died too. Some of the children her daughters left were taken by their fathers. For the remaining three orphans living with Mama Mkago, some of their paternal relatives live in the village but they do not provide help. Mama Mkago gets money for daily expenses from local brew sales and from renting the two rooms. Her husband lives in Dar es Salaam and he occasionally sends money for the household expenses. She also gets support from a daugh-ter who lives in the village. When Mama Mkago has nothing to give to the children, they get meals at their aunt's house. Mama Mkago's two sons are living in a different village but do not give any support for the orphans' care. She says: 'They do not know the pain to bear and bring up children'.

Mama Mkago did not work on her distant farm because she had to care for her daughter, who died in February 2005. She had a complicated pregnancy with frequent illness but people suspect she died of AIDS because she was living with a man known to be HIV/AIDS-infected. Though Mama Mkago makes and sells local brew, she feels that this work should be done by younger women. She is only doing it for the orphans. They are often suspended from school for lack of some of the basic requirements. They are not exempted from these requirements, even though the school knows that they are orphans.

income-generating activities that are difficult to perform at their age. For instance, to make local brew takes three working days. As women grow older their physical capacity to work declines, but many have to keep on working to provide for the orphans. Most of the income-earning activities they pursue depend on their declining physical strength and do not yield financial security, leaving them unable to meet all the expenses for food, medical care and education.

5.2.2 Impact on financial resources

Illness always places a financial burden on families and has a substantial impact on poor households. Financial resources include cash and other liquid resources such as savings, credit, remittances and pensions, which are essential to people's livelihoods. When the household has an AIDS patient, the financial burden becomes enormous as a result of direct costs of care and treatment and the disruption of regular income due to care-giving responsibilities. Households that care for AIDS patients and those who experienced deaths due to AIDS recall spending between

TShs. 3,000 and 400,000 per months on medical expenses with an average of TShs. 27,186 per month. This figure is higher than the average (TShs. 11,156) household medical expenses in rural areas in Tanzania (URT, 2002). Increased medical expenses can be attributed to prolonged illnesses. The figures do not reflect other expenses related to care, such as food supplies and consumables like soap and kerosene. The costs of care are much higher if these are taken into consideration as well. Increased medical and health care for households caring for AIDS patients made some of them unable to meet those costs.

Privatization of health care has reduced access to medical and health care. Most of the households caring for AIDS patients cannot afford to pay for these services. Though it has been declared nationally that all HIV/AIDS patients are eligible for free treatment, most people have not tested or keep their condition secret, and are thus treated as normal patients. Those who got treatment from public dispensaries complained of the poor services offered and opted for private dispensaries. The costs at private dispensaries are so high that most low-income households are unable to pay them. There are many cases where the patients were not taken to the hospital because they lacked the money and were therefore cared for at home, only to be given self-prescribed medication, mainly painkillers. Depending on what the family believed to be the cause of the illness, some resorted to traditional healers though the costs were equally high. Many households used their savings to cater for medical care, funeral expenses and other household expenses. Those who are permanently employed by the Sugar Company got medical assistance and support during funerals. There were very few who got remittances to attend the sick or pay for funerals. At the same time, remittances expected from young adults are lost when they die of AIDS, depriving households of an important source of income.

To maintain the declining income due to increased medical and other household expenses, households that had sick people got cash from various sources as shown in Table 5.11. Most of the respondents reported using their own savings to bear the cost of medical treatment and funerals. When they had no more money, they resorted to selling assets such as furniture, a radio, bicycles, and livestock such as pig and chicken. Other households sold food stocks, which endangers their food security.

Because of the increasing demands posed by care, household members, particularly women, are eventually unable to work in the fields and in other non-farm activities. This leads to a loss of productivity and income. Focused group discussions (FGD 8, see Table 3.2) revealed that another indirect financial loss induced by HIV/AIDS is lack of access to credits as affected individuals and households are regarded as less credit-worthy because members of HIV/AIDS-affected households are unable to work. In case they are able to get a loan, most of it will be used for health care and not for investing in productive activities, which creates a problem of paying back.

Table 5.11. Sources of cash to cover medical expenses (N=45).

Sources	Frequency	Percentage
Own savings	24	53.3
Relatives and friends	4	8.9
Crop sales	7	15.6
Sale of other assets	5	11.1
Employer	3	6.7
Causal work	1	2.2
Petty businesses	1	2.2
Total	45	100.0

Source: Household survey, 2005.

5.2.3 Impacts on physical and natural assets

Since costs of medical treatment for AIDS patients are high and households lack cash, some resorted to distress sales of assets. About 35 percent of HIV/AIDS-affected households reported to have sold their assets during the past five years. Among the commonly assets sold were bicycles which are important means of transportation in the area. Many people use bicycles to avoid bus fares, and use the money thus saved for other purposes. Distress sale of items usually fetches very low prices since those buying from such households take advantage of their problems and offer them the lowest price possible. Once households exhaust their productive assets, it is unlikely that they can recover and rebuild their livelihoods. There were few cases of land sale because many people have no rights on the land they are farming on. They mostly farm on hired plots.

5.2.4 HIV/AIDS impacts on livelihood activities

As a result of HIV/AIDS, direct loss of human capital, diversion of resources and income to medical care and caring activities and forced disposal of productive assets to pay for medical care and funerals, are having a critical impact on the activities on which rural families depend for their livelihood. Premature death of young adults, force young children become household heads without proper knowledge on how to make a living. Agricultural knowledge and entrepreneurial skills are not passed from parents to children, leaving the younger generation not well prepared to engage in farming and other livelihood activities, as is demonstrated by the case of Naomi

(Case 5.1). Loss of intergenerational transfer of knowledge compromises livelihood security and renders households' vulnerable to HIV/AIDS impacts.

Despite diversification of rural livelihood activities, the most prominent activity in the area is farming. Apart from farming other income-generating activities are marketing of crops, gardening, beer brewing, food vending, daily casual piecework, petty trade and formal employment with the Sugar Company and other service institutions in the village. The possibility to venture into non-farm income-generating activities depends on the resource base of the households involved. From the Focus Group Discussions (FGD 2, see Table 3.2) it became apparent that most of the households have not sufficient money and other inputs to invest in farming and other activities because of widespread poverty. The situation is worse for HIV/AIDS-affected households. For households caring for AIDS patients, their involvement in income-earning activities becomes constrained, due to less available active labour, cash and time to invest in those activities. Farming depends on household labour and often labour demands are concentrated in specific periods of the year. In case of sickness, most of the farm operations cannot be done on time which causes poor harvests. Livestock-keeping is also affected because households are forced to sell the animals to meet medical and other care-related costs. Some households involved in the study sold livestock such as pig, goats and chicken to meet medical and funeral expenses. HIV/AIDS-affected households have no means to get capital investment for business, as demonstrated by Naomi (Case 5.1). As a consequence, HIV/AIDS-affected households have few alternatives to supplement the low income or replenish what has been used.

HIV/AIDS-affected households shift from distant farming to home-based, small-scale income-generating activities like home-gardening, selling vegetables, charcoal and rice buns, and also local brew-making (see Cases 5.4, 5.5 and 5.7). Home gardens are located close to the house, which makes it convenient to combine working in the garden and looking after the sick. Mainly vegetables are grown, such as sweet potato, pumpkin, amarathus and okra. The vegetables are for home consumption, only the surplus – if any – is sold. If patients are bedridden, the care demands increase such that working for income becomes impossible. Those who are the sole caregivers to terminally ill persons cannot engage in income-generating activities, resulting in an overall decrease of income. Rich households use hired labour to work in their fields. For poor households this is not an option, since most of them cannot afford to pay wages. There are also some non-farm activities that are difficult for affected households to engage in, for example local brewing. Also because of stigma, the villagers are reluctant to buy items prepared and sold by those who are known to be HIV/AIDS-afflicted. These attitudes limit affected households' income-earning capacity.

5.3 Social and moral aspects of HIV/AIDS impacts on the household

5.3.1 Family-based care

Because of the moral contents in family relationships, household members and kin function as a resort for social support (Pennartz & Niehof, 1999). Care-giving requires significant levels of effort and resources within the household. Caring for AIDS-patients differs from caring people suffering from other diseases, because of the complex nature of the affliction, as manifested in the various ways in which health is affected, and the long duration, stigma (Radstake, 2000) and incurability (Simon *et al.*, 2006; Bruce *et al.*, 2000). The intensity of the required care varies, depending on whether the person is mobile or bedridden. If the AIDS-patient stays at home and is confined to bed, the caregiver(s) may need to be full-time available. Although care covers a range of services and activities, in the study area care was mainly understood as the provision of instrumental care. For a bedridden family member this may involve bathing and cleaning up, hand-feeding for those too sick to feed themselves, washing clothes, toilet assistance, turning the sick to avoid bedsores, obtaining and preparing meals, purchasing and administering drugs. Additionally, it may require accompanying the patient to the hospital, bringing food to the hospital and supplementing nursing care. In addition to all these households members have to engage in activities to earn income for household survival needs and cater for additional care demands.

Household financial resources determine the level and quality of care provided. Care-related expenses include travel to and from the hospital, purchase of medicines or treatments, purchase of other consumables such as soap, kerosene, sugar and special diets. Seven out of the 15 case studies concern households with chronically ill household members and are suspected AIDS-cases. In six out of these seven cases (Cases 5.4, 5.5, 5.7, 6.1, 6.2 and 7.2) the households are struggling to provide adequate care in a situation of dwindling resources. Lack of skills and knowledge (competence) on handling AIDS-patients also hinders provision of adequate care. These issues are illustrated by the following case.

As illustrated by the case of Mama Oliva, caring presents an economic and emotional drain to the caregiver who also runs the risk of contracting HIV infection. Home care puts caregivers at risk of infection, because they may nurse the sick without protecting themselves and taking precautions. Caregivers do not seem to recognize the importance of such measures. Denial may also prevent caregivers, especially parents, from taking necessary precautions. When parents do not accept the child's HIV-status, they may not comply with the prescribed ways to handle such patients.

Although proximity and the daily sharing among people belonging to one household reinforce their awareness of mutual moral obligations (Pennartz & Niehof, 1999), care tasks can be performed by persons beyond the household, like relatives. People are expected to care for sick relatives, but the evidence provided by ten HIV/AIDS-affected case studies shows otherwise. The fact that those affected or their caregivers do not inform relatives about the true nature of the illness is one explanation. Additionally, provision of care requires resources, notably money. Interviews in case studies and with key informants showed that moral and emotional support is given but not money. Lack of money was reported to be an important constraint to care for the sick. Households may have good intentions to provide care to ill relatives but they may lack the means to do so.

Care by parents is inspired by love for their children and is provided in a context of reciprocity between the generations that extends over the life course. The quality of the relationship involved and reciprocal obligations influence care. Mama Oliva (Case 5.4) nurses her daughter at a time when she could have expected her daughter to provide support to her. From Mama Oliva's complaints, it is clear that she realizes that her expectations were defeated. AIDS creates care demands and is likely to kill young adults before they can reciprocate to their parents and other family members. Moreover, as was pointed out during focus group discussion (FGD 8, see Table 3.2), the fact that AIDS is known to be fatal implies that the patient cannot return the favour in the future. The perceived incurability of AIDS makes people feel that it is pointless to offer good quality care at the expense of your resources. HIV/AIDS-related stigma also affects care provision to affected individuals and households.

5.3.2 HIV/AIDS stigma

HIV/AIDS-related stigma influences care for affected individuals by the family and other community members, and also negatively affects preventive actions like HIV-testing. In the study area, HIV/AIDS is commonly referred to as the modern sickness (*ugonjwa wa kisasa*). Different metaphors are used to explain the pandemic such as electric shock (*umeme*), implying that once you have it you are gone because usually an electric shock kills instantly. Another notion is a network (*mtandao*), meaning that those infected are likely to spread the infection to others. HIV/AIDS is also referred to as an insect (*mdudu*), meaning that those affected can bite others and transmit the infection. All these metaphors describe the nature of the disease and stigmatize those affected. People living with HIV/AIDS are subject to name calling and labeling, like 'a dead person to be' or a 'moving skeleton'.

Regardless of how people become infected with HIV, the assumption is that the infection is the result of morally questionable behaviour. It is often presumed that

Case 5.4. Mama Oliva: caring for an AIDS patient.

Mama Oliva (63) is living with her two sons in a two-room house. Her sons have casual jobs in the village, and there are times they are out of work altogether. Mama Oliva has a vegetable garden from which she gets the vegetables for family consumption and for sale. Her daughter who had been living in the village is sick and had to move to her mother's house for care. The daughter was living with a married man, who has not visited her since she moved to her mother's house. She had twins who died a year ago. Mama Oliva did not tell her neighbours that her daughter moved in. Mama Oliva took her daughter to the hospital where she was diagnosed with low blood pressure and prolonged constipation. Mama Oliva never mentioned HIV/AIDS. For the first three months Mama Oliva was able to work in her garden, but as her daughter's condition got worse, she was barely able to do so. First, for a few days a week she was able to buy and sell vegetables, in front of her house. But when her daughter became bedridden, she had to stop doing this too; she now spends most of her time attending to her.

Even without a sick person in the household, Mama Oliva could not save money from the vegetable sales, because whatever she earned was used for daily household expenses. Because of lack of money, she could not take her daugh-ter to be admitted to the hospital. Mama Oliva complained several times of a lack of money to buy the necessary items and drugs. Her sister, who lives in Dar es Salaam, promised to send money for medical expenses but did not do so. The income from the two sons is not steady and not enough to cover the increasing health care costs. The boys resorted to using their meager income for eating outside. Several times I passed by their house and found the patient alone in the house, because Mama Oliva had gone to buy food or medicine. Neighbours told me that the daughter is often left alone without the neighbours being asked to keep an eye on her.

Mama Oliva nurses her daughter without using gloves. She says she cannot use gloves on her own child and that she has no money to buy them anyway. The patient is given the same food as the other family members, though the diet is unbalanced and difficult for an invalid to take. Mama Oliva looks exhausted and tired. Mama Oliva once complained that when her daughter was well, though living in the same village, she would go for months without seeing her mother and did not provide any financial support to her mother. Now that she is sick, it is her mother she turns to. Mama Oliva spends whole days and sleepless nights attending to her. 'Basically my entire day is dominated by activities to help my daughter', Mama Oliva says. Her daughter is thankful for her mother's care, and said that her mother is the only one who helps her. Mama Oliva went to a local traditional healer and was given some medicine. She was told that her daughter has been bewitched by her co-wife. Three days after using the herbs Mama Oliva's daughter passed away. I was not in the village to attend the funeral. Mama Oliva told me that her relatives from Dar es Salaam came, financed the funeral, and gave money to go to their original home in Kigoma to report the death to other relatives. The daughter was buried in the village. The man she was once living with did not come to the burial for fear of being ac-cused of being responsible for her death. Her brother who lives away was not informed of her illness, so her death came as a surprise to him.

those living with the virus have brought disease upon themselves by having sex with many partners. Hence, HIV/AIDS becomes associated with immoral behaviour. Some perceive the disease as the penalty for sinners, for not being obedient to God. This kind of prejudice is justified by a statement like: 'What would you have done to God to deserve such a punishment'. Focus Group Discussion (FGD 9, see Table 3.2) revealed that single women in particular are subject to stigma as they are assumed to have sexual relations with many different men. Women who are known or suspected to be involved in multiple sex relations are perceived by the community as a public danger as they are likely to spread the disease. People may say: 'Be careful with that lady, she is dangerous'. These notions direct blame to people with HIV/AIDS and make assumptions made about their past sexual behaviour. Women are especially prone to this prejudice. Women experience more stigma and discrimination related to HIV/AIDS than men, because of the gendered societal perceptions on promiscuity and sexuality. It is accepted for men to have multiple sexual relationships but not for women. The masculine culture found in many parts of the country encourages men to have multiple partners. On the other hand, women are expected to be innocent, married and live with one man only, and any different behaviour subjects women to stigmatization. Because of their subordinate status in society, many women are stigmatized as the vector of HIV transmission.

Social isolation is one of the most challenging problems faced by individuals suffering from AIDS-related infections and families caring for AIDS-patients. In the household and family setting, stigma is manifested in forms of rejection and abandonment. Some of the married women who are known to be HIV/AIDS-infected are abandoned by their husbands, leaving them dependent on the often minimal support from relatives and the community (Case 5.4 and Case 6.3). It was also found that inability to contribute to the household may add to the stigma associated with HIV/AIDS. Affected persons are regarded unworthy by their family and in their community, which increases the chances of being stigmatized. Stigma is not just painful to those concerned; it may also hamper care from family members, as shown in the following short narrative which was reported during the Focus Group discussion with youth on HIV/AIDS issues:

A young HIV-positive mother had a baby by Caesarean section. When she was admitted her sister whom she was staying with and other relatives did not visit her. After being discharged from the hospital she went to live with her sister. The HIV/AIDS-positive mother was continuously crying, because she had AIDS but also because she did not get any support from her relatives. While staying with her sister, she was not given money for medical care or the food she needed. She later decided to move in with her sister's friend who sympathized with her situation.

Despite the existing awareness about HIV/AIDS transmission modes as shown in national data (see Chapter 1), in the village people could be frequently observed to put physical distance between them and persons suspected of having AIDS. Not shaking hands with or not sitting next to afflicted people, not sharing drinks at local bars and not buying local brew from those who are known or assumed to be HIV-infected are all signs of stigmatization. Refusal to buy from someone who is known to be infected can be devastating to that person's economic survival.

Hiding HIV-status forms an obstacle for prevention and treatment. People do not want to go for testing because the likely stigmatization when tested positive outweighs the perceived advantages of testing. Those who are known to be HIV-positive are an object of discussion in the community and are pointed at as being responsible for some deaths in the village. Hence, people are reluctant to disclose their HIV-positive status to try to avoid the consequences of their status becoming public knowledge. It was said during a focus group discussion (FGD 8, see Table 3.2) that those who are not tested feel that is better to remain in the dark. Fear for stigmatization makes HIV-infected individuals to forego health and medical services that could lengthen their life and improve their quality of life. Local health staff told me about a proposed test for women attending antenatal clinics in local hospitals and dispensaries deterred some of them from registering for maternal clinic visits.

During the focus group discussion on HIV/AIDS and its impacts (FGD 9, see Table 3.2), ignorance and misinformation about how HIV is transmitted and how it progresses with time were identified as the main causes of stigma. The widespread notion that once one has contracted HIV one is going to die soon contributes to deepening the stigma. Such beliefs are prevalent and hinder people's willingness to do an HIV-test. People fear that a positive test results predicts a quick death. One person who had been living with HIV/AIDS for seven years and who was open about it, said: 'Having AIDS is not the end of the world. There are misconceptions among the people that once you have it you will die the next day.' Fears of illness and death make people unwilling to know about or their health status but also make them avoid contact with people with AIDS. Some people said it is emotionally demoralising and upsetting seeing AIDS patients in their terminal stage, preventing friends and relatives to seek contact with them, unless they are very close relatives. To avoid stigma people try to find alternative explanations of their illness.

5.3.3 Secrecy and witchcraft-induced illness

As discussed above, HIV/AIDS-afflicted persons mostly prefer to remain silent about their condition for fear of bad treatment by the family and the community. It was found that other household members of the afflicted case studies seemed to be aware of the condition of their ill relative but would not tell anyone outside their household. Neighbours could be suspicious about the cause of the illness, but were never sure. During in-depth interviews some respondents (Cases 5.4, 6.1 and 6.4) maintained that their condition was due to other problems or witchcraft. Others mentioned HIV/AIDS only as a cause of death. Among seven case studies with sick persons, in only one case (Case 7.2) being HIV/AIDS-positive was explicitly admitted. Exposing one's status to a stranger is not so threatening because that would not interfere with the daily interaction with other members of the family or community. As Radstake (2000) also found, in a situation where AIDS is highly stigmatized one has to be secretive about one's condition to prevent social exclusion.

While secrecy and silence about HIV/AIDS prevail at individual and household level, people openly talk about it in public. People were heard discussing about issues related to HIV/AIDS in many informal settings, for example in a local bar or restaurant. During an interview with one of the leaders of an organization of people living with HIV/AIDS in the district (SHDEPHA$^+$), this man said that in his opinion secrecy contributes to further spread of the disease. He had made his positive HIV-status public. But people think he is cheating, because they believe people cannot be open about it and still get positive treatment from the community. People call him names, but he is standing by his decision to fight the stigma and make the community aware that there is a life with HIV. Though people are encouraged to publicly disclose their HIV/AIDS status, there is no much support for those who have done so. There is little or no treatment and support available for those who have been diagnosed positive. It is not only because of stigma but also the lack of care and treatment services that has contributed to people's reluctance to get tested. One young lady said:

> *'There is no need of knowing more about your health status if you cannot have access to drugs and other support once you are sick and not able to work.'*

People who find out that they are HIV-positive often respond by denying the diagnosis and look for alternative explanations for their illnesses. Witchcraft beliefs provide such an explanation. Many respondents attribute HIV-related signs and symptoms to traditional diseases or witchcraft. Some who have full-blown AIDS still deny it and rather say that they are bewitched. To be bewitched is not shameful. The burden of blame is then shifted to those responsible for the bewitching. People who are bewitched receive greater acceptance, better treatment, and can be open about their condition. They receive sympathy and understanding from family and community members. Although prolonged illness of household member is sometimes associated with witchcraft, there was a disagreement during a focus group discussion on HIV/AIDS issues (FGD 8, see Table 3.2) on the question of whether AIDS could be caused by witchcraft. Some said a person can be bewitched and have illness symptoms like those related to AIDS. Others objected by arguing that if someone does not like to see her/his enemy any longer, s/he will kill the person instantly and will not let him/her live and suffer from an AIDS-related prolonged illness. Because of the strength of witchcraft beliefs and the acceptability of witchcraft claims in the area, people tend to accept a diagnosis of witchcraft better than one of AIDS and opt to visit a traditional healer rather than going to the hospital for an HIV-test. Though the participants in the focus group discussion seemed to be aware that traditional healers cannot cure AIDS, people still visit them when they believe the cause of their illness to be witchcraft. Among the 12 HIV/AIDS-affected case studies, in five cases witchcraft was mentioned as the cause of their illness. I also came across several other people suffering from prolonged illness who attributed their illness to witchcraft.

5.4 Effects of HIV/AIDS on household food security

Household food security is an important livelihood outcome and an indicator of vulnerability. Many people in the study area complained about the hard economic conditions, manifested in income and food insecurity. It was found that not only HIV/AIDS influences household food security but there are other factors as well. During the focus group discussions various factors contributing to food insecurity and prolonged hunger periods in the village were identified. They included lack of resources, such as labour and cash, to invest in distant farms, low productivity in agriculture, unpredictable weather and bad harvests. Furthermore, it was said that labour is scarce due to increased illness and deaths in households, while rice – both a food and a cash crop – requires heavy labour input at specific periods, which is a problem when it is produced on distant farms. Failure to timely attend the rice farm results in low harvests, which may later cause household food insecurity.

Providing enough food becomes a problem for households when there is no longer anyone to work on the farm and or earn an income from off- and non-farm activities. The tendency to have all kinds of celebrations after the harvest forces households to spend big quantities of foods, which may result into food insecurity later. Farmers have low negotiation power when selling their crops to traders who buy on-farm. During the harvest season businessmen (traders) from different parts of the country, especially Pemba, buy paddy at relatively low prices as compared to those in urban markets. The price of a hundred kilogram of paddy is between TShs. 15,000 and 18,000 when sold on-farm, but when sold in the urban market or off-season can reach TShs. 30,000. Because of the high cost of transporting the paddy from the distant farms, people opt to sell their produce on-farm and keep a few bags they can afford to transport themselves, which may not be enough for the whole year.

Most households in the village experience food shortages between November and March, a period is commonly known in the area as *masika*. According to the participants in the Focus Group Discussion 1 and 2 (see Table 3.2), the community knows there is widespread food insecurity when the following happens:

- Increased number of people engaged in daily wage activities.
- Increased marital problems, because women may be forced to engage in paid sex to buy food for the family.
- Low school attendance of children.
- Reduced quantity and quality of meals.
- Reduced paddy quantities for sun-drying.
- Increased number of people who collect rice grains from the rice-milling machine.
- Increased purchases of grain or flour from the shops.
- Increased visits by children (especially during meal times) to households known to have food.

As indicated in Table 5.12, more than 30 percent of the respondents in the survey could be categorized as food insecure.

5.4.1 Empirical statistical analysis

At first, a bivariate analysis was used to determine the association between food security, HIV/AIDS status and socio-economic status. The results produced a statistically significant association between food security and socio-economic status (Table 5.12) but not between food security and HIV/AIDS status (Table 5.13).

To increase the statistical power multivariate analysis was performed between food security and other explanatory variables. Ordinal regression was used because it

Table 5.12. Household food security status by socio-economic status (N=180).

Food security status	Socio-economic status						Total	
	Poor		Moderately poor		Well off			
	(N)	Percent	(N)	Percent	(N)	Percent	(N)	Percent
Food secure	6	14.6	29	23.3	11	73.4	46	25.6
Moderately food insecure	22	53.7	55	44.4	2	13.3	79	43.9
Food insecure	13	31.7	40	32.3	2	13.3	55	30.5
Total	41	100	124	100	15	100	180	100

$\chi 2$= 21.221, p=0.000.
Source: Household survey, 2005.

Table 5.13. Household HIV/AIDS status by food security status (N=180).

HIV/AIDS	Food security status							
	Food secure		Moderately food insecure		Food insecure		Total	
	(N)	Percent	(N)	Percent	(N)	Percent	(N)	Percent
Affected	5	16.3	17	56.7	8	27.0	30	16.7
Non-affected	41	27.3	62	41.3	47	31.4	150	83.3
Total	46	25.6	79	44.0	55	30.4	180	100

$\chi 2$= 2.630, p=0.268.
Source: Household survey, 2005.

retains the ranking order within the dependent variable. Explanatory variables included age, household headship, education level, marital status, dependency ratio, land ownership, income, sale of labour, membership in groups, presence of persons with chronic illnesses, experience of death in the household, support in times of illnesses, support in times of food shortages. At first, the food security total score as discussed in Chapter 3 was used but the differences between the scores ranging from 5 to 15 were too small to yield significant results. Therefore, the scores were combined into the three categories of food insecure (score 5-10), moderately food insecure (score 11-14) and food secure (score 15).

HIV/AIDS-affected as defined in the study (see Chapter 3) did not produce significant effects (see Appendix 1). This may be because of difficulties to observe impacts when households with chronically ill members, those that experienced death and those that took in orphans, are lumped together. Households with orphans could be relatively food secure because, depending on the gender, age and the number of orphans taken in, the intake of orphans may have increased their labour potential, thereby enhancing food security. It might also be that they were relatively well-off before the orphans joined their household. So, if any, the effect of taking orphans would be positive, while the effect of the presence of persons with prolonged illnesses who are unable to work can be assumed to be negative. The presence of persons with prolonged illnesses is often taken as a proxy for HIV/AIDS-status. We took the reported prolonged illnesses of tuberculosis, pneumonia or chronic malaria to be indicative of AIDS. As explained in Section 5.2.1, 45 households had people with prolonged illness, out of which 15 households were in the HIV/AIDS-affected group as defined in study. These 45 households were included in the analysis. Prolonged illnesses, whether or not caused by HIV/AIDS, was found to have a significant effect on household food security. Unlike what was done in Table 5.12, for this analysis the estimated total household income was taken as a proxy for household economic status. The results of the analysis are presented in Table 5.14.

The sex of the household head is significantly related to food security, confirming that male-headed households tend to have more resources than female-headed ones, which contributes to the food security. Also being married, though not highly significantly, contributes to food security. Although the dependency ratio has no significant influence on household food security, Table 5.9 showed that more women-headed households (43.2%) than male-headed households (30.7%) have high effective dependency ratios. Households with a high dependency ratio are likely to be more food insecure because of the unfavourable ratio between working and non-working members who all have to be fed. The table shows the expected negative relationship between dependency ratio and food security, but it is not significant. The sale of labour is positively related to household food security. Households with high number of adults who are physically-fit are likely to sell their labour to earn money for food. Sale of labour was identified as one means to get income for the household as reported by almost 49 percent of the respondents. People in the area can get casual jobs to work in the Sugarcane Company estate or get employed by sugarcane farmers.

Table 5.14. Factors influencing household food security (N=180).

Explanatory variables	B-coefficient	Standaard error
Age (years)	0.0028323	0.0115162
Household headship (1=male)	1.289767**	0.5796451
Education level (1=educated)	-0.1118856	0.3894887
Effective dependency ratio	-0.1615567	0.2062981
Marital status (1=married)	0.93242*	0.4964907
No. of people with chronic illnesses	-0.578521**	0.2865976
Death/s in the household (1=yes)	-0.0450753	0.3376652
Estimated household annual income (Tshs)	8.25e-07***	2.95e-07
Land ownership (1=yes)	0.23507	0.3201263
Sale of labour (1=yes)	1.717412***	0.3410562
Group membership (1=yes)	0.2159307	0.3105925
Support during illness (1=yes)	0.1164455	0.5883534
Support during food shortage (1=yes)	0.1415803	0.4080352

LR Chi^2 (13) = 58.49
Prob > Chi^2 = 0.000
Pseudo R^2 = 0.1515
Log likelihood = -163.77823
*p<0.10, **p<0.05 and ***p<0.01.
Source: Household Survey, 2005.

As could be expected, the number of people with prolonged illnesses in the household is negatively and significantly related to food security. Persons suffering from prolonged illness in the household increase its effective dependency ratio. In the survey, HIV/AIDS-affected household appeared to have relatively higher (40%) effective dependency ratio than non-affected households (32%), though the difference is not significant (see Table 5.8). As Christiaensen & Subbarao (2004) argued, the higher the dependency ratio the more the household is vulnerable to poverty. Group membership and support in case of illness and food shortage relate positively – though not significantly – to food security. This finding may indicate the lack or only limited support households get from their relatives, friends and neighbours in case of those problems, even those households that need it most. Community groups in the village do not provide support in case of food shortage and but only occasionally provide support in case of illness.

Although most of households in the village face either seasonal or chronic food insecurity, poor are especially vulnerable. During the Focus Group Discussion 5 (see Table 3.2), it was reported that poor households are likely to face food shortage for longer periods in a year. Income is significantly positively related to food security, as expected. It was interesting to note that six poor households are food secure. However, three of them are single-person households who have to provide food for just one person. Even if they do not have food stocks of their own they can access food from local food vendors or restaurants, whether or not on credit.

5.4.2 Qualitative analysis

Chronic illnesses of household members not only reduce food production, but also the household's capacity to generate income to purchase food. This is illustrated by Case 5.5.

The cumulative impacts of prolonged illness on food production and food access have adverse effects on overall household food security, as is illustrated by Mama Zalima's case and other case studies (Cases 5.7, 6.1, 6.3 and 7.2). The resources needed for food production are severely eroded by having an AIDS patient in the household. Especially farming on distant farms becomes difficult in households with sick people. Cases 5.7 and 7.2 show how illness prevents the male adult household member from having a casual job, which results in food shortages. Use of hired labour for the farming plots is not feasible for poor households. Household income is reduced and without any external financial assistance the food intake of the household members will decline. Reduced food intake may also affect the health of non-affected members. Mama Zalima gets occasional income from brewing activities. Though local brew-making is undertaken by many women in the area, it yields low profits and is quite risky. Another study conducted in Tanzania showed the risks associated with brewing. Since the majority of beer sellers are women and their main customers are men, women may be at increased risk of offering or being forced to have sex with their customers in order to sell their beer (Mackay, 2003), which increases their susceptibility to HIV infection.

Coping with food insecurity: a stone in the cooking pot

Households faced with food shortages adopt a variety of coping mechanisms. Results from the focus group discussions and case studies offer insights into how households cope with food insecurity. Daily causal labour on a piecework basis is practiced by many households and involves working for others in the fields, often in exchange for cash. This is a common response for households in the area, including affected households, provided there are other members in the household who can work.

Case 5.5. Mama Zalima: HIV/AIDS-affected, food insecure.

In the shade I met Mama Zalima who lives in a single room with her sister and two children, a girl (11) and a boy (8). Her sister did not want to talk to me in all four interviews I had with Mama Zalima. They both came to the village in 1995. Mama Zalima's husband, who worked as a seasonal labourer in sugar plantations, left her and went back to Iringa in 2001. Then her sister joined Mama Zalima's household. Mama Zalima is a farmer, but she also sells local brew in the nearby local bar. They have a rice farm in Lwegama and the sisters used to take It in turns to go there because one of them had to stay with the school-going children. Her sister has been suffering from TB for the past two years. The nurse responsible for community-based care told me she has AIDS, but Mama Zalima did not mention this. Her sister used to get medication from the local dispensary and a community-based team in the village. She no longer wants to go to a local public dispensary alleging that she was mistreated and they did not prescribe the proper medica-tion. Eventually, she went to a traditional healer who gave her traditional medicines, which she is no longer taking. Mama Zalima said even after prolonged use of traditional medicines her sister has not been cured.

The previous season they harvested ten bags of rice. At the time of interview they had no stock left and were buying everything from the shops. 'It is not easy to have food stocks for the whole year with all these problems', Mama Zalima says. During her sister's illness she had to sell six bags of rice to cover the medical expenses. During her sister's Illness Mama Zalima could not engage in income-generating activities and did not get any financial assistance. Their house-mates took her sister to the hospital but didn't give them money because they also had none. Mama Zalima says: 'Our life was miserable but we survived'. Her sister's illness has made her bankrupt and she will have to start all over again. 'Our life will never be the same. Imagine, my sister used to do her own business and contribute to household income but now she entirely relies on me'. She wanted to ask for assistance from the village but her sister prevented her from doing so, claiming that people would laugh at them. Despite all these problems, Mama Zalima has to make cash con-tributions for the construction of the local school. She is not a member of any group, because she cannot pay the fees and other contributions. All the money she gets from her brewing is used for family needs and her sister's medical ex-penses.

They have not planted anything this season because they have no money to invest in farming and Mama Zalima cannot go to the farm since she has to be at home to look after her sister and the children. She cannot afford to hire people to work on their plot. During those times when her sister feels well she makes and sells local brew, though the business is risky. Sometimes the brew does not mature well and there's a risk of losing all the money invested. On aver-age you need to invest about TShs. 12,000 to realize a profit of about TShs. 3,000. Some clients take the brew on credit. When Mama Zalima does not get enough money from brewing, their daily food becomes a problem. They fre-quently skip meals unless she is able to get food loans from the shops, which is difficult since she still has debts to pay. One day I found her walking about aimlessly. When I asked her what was the matter, she told me: 'We have nothing for food today. I am just roaming about, I might be lucky to get some money to buy food'.

Households, in which adults, who could have worked, are sick, face severe food shortages.

Reducing the quality and quantity of food intake is another response to food insecurity. During Focus Group Discussion 2 (see Table 3.2) it became apparent that households facing food shortages live on fewer meals than normal. When there is enough food, most people prefer three rice meals a day, but when they start experiencing food shortage they resort to less preferred foods such as maize meal and wild vegetables. In very critical situations people just have to go on one meal a day or none at all. Children are likely to beg or play around households known to have enough food, hoping to be invited for meals. Girls can ask for domestic work to get food in return, while boys may resort to stealing from people's home or farms.

Gender plays a key role in household food security and its ability to cope with food shortages. Both men and women take part in on-farm food production activities, but after harvest the men generally decide on the use of harvested crop. Rice is both a cash and food crop in the area, so there are competing interests in its use. Since men's decisions prevail, much of the harvest ends up being sold, leaving the households with little or no food to take them through the year. In case of food shortage, women have to seek for means to get food. Some do so by trying to engage themselves in income-generating activities, such as making local brew, food vending and home-based businesses like selling charcoal or running a small kiosk that sells basic household necessities, but this is not easy. Focus Group Discussion 2 (see Table 3.2) disclosed that in times of food insecurity, women may resort to paid sex to be able to buy food for their family, which increases the risk of HIV-infection, especially since they do so unprotected. Women pointed out that it is better to buy food with the little money they have than buying a condom. In village shops, a pack of three condoms costs TShs. 100, enough to buy relish to go with the rice or maize meal. Further probing during the focused group discussions yielded an interesting but sad finding. Participants pointed out that in case of severe food shortage a woman may put a stone in a cooking pot and put it on the fire, to let the children think that there is something cooking. So the children will play around, thinking there will be something to eat later on. While the stone is cooking the woman will have time to search for food. This shows how desperate women can be in times of food shortage.

5.5 AIDS and livelihood vulnerability

Household's ability to access food through various means and ability to cope with food shortages and sicknesses is used as an indicator of vulnerability. Although HIV/AIDS affects people from all socio-economic strata, Cases 5.6 and 5.7 indicate

Case 5.6. Hawa: HIV/AIDS-affected, coping sustainably with AIDS impacts.

Hawa (38) is married as a second wife to a famous businessman in the area. She is living with two other relatives who came to seek help from her. She is a successful farmer who hires labour to work in her farm and can harvest up to 1,000 bags of rice per season. She stocks and sells the rice In the off-season. She also has a hardware shop in the village. Her father is a popular politician in the district. She has been treated in Dar es Salaam for her skin condition. When she was seriously ill, her father hired a car and took her to Ifakara Hospital and later to the Aga Khan Hospital in Dar es Salaam. She did not tell me that she has AIDS but people told me she is currently living on ARVs. Hawa gets care from the relatives she is living with. Despite her condition, she is involved in many women's organizations in the district and in the village and is a leader of one of them.

Case 5.7. Mr. Kanyango: poor, inability to cope with AIDS impacts.

Mr. Kanyango has two wives who are both from the same region. He inherited the second wife from an uncle who passed away in 1997. The first wife has four children and the second a one-year-old daughter. Mr. Kanyango was invited by his uncle in 1992 to come and work at the Sugar Company as a casual labourer. Since last year he had been suffering from TB and skin infections. He was once admitted to the hospital. To meet the expenses the first wife decided to sell a coffee table, then the rice they had in stock, and finally a bicycle. The latter was sold at a very low price. Some friends visited him while he was in hospital but did not give him any money. The first wife looked after him when he was in the hospital, the second wife ran the home.

Mr. Kanyango's household did not do any farming in the season at the time of the interview, because they had no money to hire a plot nearby and Mr. Kanyango's condition prevented him from working on the distant farm. Mr. Kanyago says that if he gets well, he will look for a job in the Sugar Company again. He acknowledges that their lives have changed since he started getting sick and at times they can only afford one meal a day. The second wife used to sell sorghum porridge in front of their house, but now she is using the business capital to buy medicines. The wives were involved in local brewing but Mr. Kanyango stopped them, claiming that they would become prostitutes. He uses to beat his wives, not bothering about how they were treated for their injuries. One of the wives said: 'We are just fed up by his behaviour'. He prevented them from doing business but cannot provide for the family himself. He has even re-stricted his wives from visiting some of their friends.

that its impacts disproportionately affect those who have the fewest economic and social resources, although the survey data do not confirm this (Table 5.13). Out 12 HIV/AIDS-affected cases (see Table 3.4) seven were in difficult circumstances even before they experienced AIDS.

HIV/AIDS intensifies the existing rural problems by contributing to a complex set of interlocking vulnerabilities. Poverty was mentioned as the main problem in the study area of both HIV/AIDS-affected and non-affected households. The evidence provided by Hawa (Case 5.6) and Mr. Kanyango (Case 5.7) shows that the initial asset base prior to infection determines the possibility to get proper medical attention and cope with other HIV/AIDS impacts. Unlike many others, Hawa (Case 5.6) is able to cope with labour shortages. The relatives who are living with her provide care when needed. She is able to continue farming and maintain her production level because she can afford treatment and is able to hire labourers to work on her farm. As shown by the case of Mr. Kanyango (Case. 5.7), for poor people relying on daily wages the situation is different. The household was deprived of income because of the breadwinner's illness. The sale of assets and food stores to meet medical costs left the household food insecure, with few resources to support their livelihood.

Inability to provide for the household disempowers men, and – as is shown in the case of Mr. Kanyango (Case 5.7) – may induce them to resort to violence to reassert their authority. Denying women the opportunity to take part in income-generating activities limits their livelihood options and increases their economic dependence on men. Mr. Kanyango's ban on his wives' brewing initiative, which he claimed would lead to extra-marital affairs, was a way of blaming them for his HIV/AIDS-status. He was using them as scapegoats. Violence may increase non-infected women's susceptibility to HIV, because they may be forced to have unsafe sex.

The presence of multiple sources of stress in the area, such as food and income insecurity, lack of land, and disruption of social networks by migration and distant farming, exacerbate the problems of AIDS. They contribute to poverty and make HIV/AIDS-affected households unable to respond to HIV/AIDS-impacts. Income diverted to medical care make households unable to hire labour and invest in food production, while sale of food stocks to get money for health care makes them food insecure. Some of HIV/AIDS impacts resemble those of other socio-economic problems experienced by non-affected households. The study area has experienced more than one shock and the following case studies show how also non-HIV/AIDS affected households are struggling to make ends meet.

Mama Wawili's case (Case 5.8) demonstrates that also non-HIV/AIDS-affected poor households experience difficulties in dealing with shocks. Women who are deserted

Case 5.8. Mama Wawili: poor household, non-HIV/AIDS affected.

Mama Wawili is aged 26 and has four children, two pairs of twins. The older twins are in class three and the younger twins were born at the time of the interviews. Mama Wawili lives with her mother who helps her look after the children. The twins are from different fathers who do not provide any support to the family. She told me that she did not plan to have another baby but got pregnant as she was trying to make her living. Mama Wawili delivered her last babies at home, despite the advice she was given during the antenatal clinic visits, because she could not afford to pay for the delivery charges in KI Hospital. Two days after Mama Wawili delivered her babies her mother had to leave for their distant farm to work on the rice-fields. At home, Mama Wawili had to struggle on her own. I once found her very weak and she told me she just had porridge, and that was all they had. Her older twins were roaming from one house to another asking for food. She got some money from selling the bananas she had harvested from the few plants in her compound. She told me her mother had left her with very little, because they had to use the money they had to hire a tractor for ploughing.

When the babies were one-and-a-half months old, she joined her mother on the farm, but unfortunately the babies got malaria and diarrhoea which forced her to go back to the village. She left her mother to work alone in the field. The situation in the rice field is unhealthy because of the high probability of contracting water-borne infections and malaria. The children were treated at the local dispensary. She could not go to the field again and she was not sure if her mother would manage to weed the entire plot without her assistance. They could not hire labourers because they had no money to pay them. Her mother was sometimes forced to work on other people's farms to earn some money to buy daily necessities while staying on the farm.

by their partners are left to struggle and fend for their family on their own. Distant farming requires high investments in terms of cash and time which most poor households do not have. In spite of the efforts of distant farmers, a good harvest is not guaranteed not only because of shortage of labour but also because of unreliable climatic conditions. Distant-farming poor households are at risk of food insecurity. The difference between affected and non-affected households is that HIV/AIDS kills productive adults who cannot be replaced, thereby undermining household livelihoods irreversibly. Mama Wawili's mother was able to continue working on the field. She did not have to stay at home with her daughter as is the case with many households with AIDS patients. Case 5.9 presents another illustration of the problems involved in distant farming.

Case 5.9. Zakia: effects of distant farming.

Zakia is a girl of 13 living with her grandmother. Her parents live in another district with their other six children. Zakia does not want to stay with her parents, because they spend most of their time in the field and she cannot go to school there. In the village she is able to attend a special primary school program for those who are beyond school age (MEMKWA). She only goes with her grandmother to the distant farm during the school holidays. When she went back recently, her grandmother gave her only TShs. 1,000, to buy relish to go with the maize meal. She was left with about three kilograms of maize flour. Zakia does not know when her grandmother, who had been away for three months at the time of the interview, will come back. Zakia's school attendance is sporadic. Because she has no food, she goes around peoples' houses in search of housework in return for food. Usually she is asked to wash the dishes, clean the house or baby-sit. Later on, she moved from her grandmother's house to a family that has taken her as a domestic helper. She no longer goes to school. She did not tell me, but her neighbour confided to me that she even had to engage in sex in exchange for food.

Zakia's situation exemplifies how land shortage in the village impacts on household members and increases the vulnerability of children. During the farming season most of the school-going children are left in the village when their parents and other adults go to the distant farms. These children are left to fend for themselves. As these children are not attending school, they are likely to become drop-outs. Distant farming increases a household's vulnerability and jeopardizes the children's future.

5.6 Discussion and conclusions

The HIV/AIDS pandemic affects different households in different ways and produces a variety of coping strategies. Although the impact of AIDS on individuals and families varies some general conclusions can been drawn. The evidence presented in this chapter, especially that from the qualitative data, describes HIV/AIDS-impacts on households and their livelihoods and the variety of ways in which households deal with these. The mortality and morbidity associated with AIDS have significant impacts on household resources and assets. Changes in household composition and individual roles are among the notable effects brought about by HIV/AIDS epidemic. The prolonged illness of a household member drains income and assets. Loss of assets and income during AIDS morbidity and mortality has been found to be major factor contributing to households' poverty and vulnerability. Loss of labour time because AIDS diverts time from productive activities to care provision, has the same effect.

The fact that HIV/AIDS affects the adult, prime-age population significantly intensifies the impact of the disease on household human capital. Due to AIDS mortality the skills on farming and other livelihood activities of the adult generation are lost for the younger generation, thereby undermining the sustainability of the livelihood prospects of the ones left behind. This applies especially to orphans. AIDS-orphans (Cases 5.1 and 5.2) were found to be vulnerable because they get no substantial assistance from the extended family; they lack cash income and other resources to manage their lives. Inability to attend school shows the long-term effect of the pandemic on future generations in terms of educational status and livelihood options.

Men and women experience HIV/AIDS impacts differently. Evidence from this study indicates that the impacts of HIV/AIDS are more critical for women than men. Socio-economic factors and cultural values place men in a more favourable position for coping with the impacts. In their roles as mothers and care providers, women are mainly responsible for taking care of HIV/AIDS patients in the home and for fostering AIDS-orphans, in addition to other productive and domestic tasks. Although men do help, women bear most of the burden of nursing sick household members. HIV/AIDS increases women's workload as they are forced to pursue both productive activities and meet the increasing care demands induced by AIDS-illnesses. When women fall ill they are likely to be abandoned by their partners while still having to look after children and not receiving the care they need (see Case 6.3). Care-giving falls disproportionably on women, especially elderly women, who have to do so with minimal resources. Caregivers are at risk of getting infected themselves, because of lack of knowledge on nursing AIDS-patients and lack of cash to buy protective gloves. Denial of positive HIV-status was found to be an obstacle to adequate prevention and care. HIV/AIDS is changing parents' expectations of support from their children in old age because it attacks at a critical age. HIV/AIDS-affected people can no longer provide for their parents but require care from them instead and also leave their children behind to be cared for. However, elderly people's reduced physical and financial capacities hinder their ability to provide care to their orphaned grandchildren.

Stigmatization because of HIV/AIDS is a problem for both affected men and women, but due to socio-cultural factors women are likely to be stigmatized more. This situation emanates from women's inferior position in the society. Fear of the reaction of the community and unavailability of support services for those affected deter people from taking an HIV-test and disclose their positive HIV-status. HIV/AIDS-related stigma not only affects people whom it is directed against, it also harms the wider population by limiting health seeking behaviour and frustrating efforts to fight against HIV/AIDS. Behavioural mechanisms such as denial and secrecy were found to be based on fear for stigma and rejection.

The quantitative findings on the determinants of food security generally affirm previous findings that health status, income and headship are powerful predictor of household food security. It is shown that households with adult members suffering from prolonged illnesses are food insecure. HIV/AIDS-affected households in the study reported lack of adequate food and income to buy food as a major problem. Such households do not have labour and cash resources for own food production. Food access is affected through declining income to purchase food. Food insecurity may force individuals to adopt livelihood strategies that may lead to greater susceptibility to HIV. In this, women are more at risk, because they are held responsible for ensuring there is enough food in the household. The impacts of HIV/AIDS on food security observed in this study are consistent with to what has been reported in other African studies (Wiegers *et al.*, 2006; Loevinsohn & Gillespie, 2003). In the study area, HIV/AIDS exacerbates household food insecurity and poverty, interacting with other factors such as distant farming, unemployment, unreliable weather and poor marketing structures.

A household's ability to offset the impacts of HIV/AIDS depends on its assets-base, its capacity to re-organize household resources, and its access to the resources of the extended family. The severity of the impacts is likely to vary according to economic status of the household, with poorer households suffering more than less poor households. Households that are rich in terms of economic and social resources (cf. Case 5.6) are better able to deal with HIV/AIDS-effects than poor households who sometimes have to adopt responses that threaten their livelihood (as in Cases 5.5 and 5.7). Many of those are likely to get trapped in downward spiral of poverty. Rugalema (2000) and De Waal & Tumushabe (2003) also suggest that HIV/AIDS-affected households never fully cope, since they cannot return to their previous situation and cannot escape the longer-term downward trend of food insecurity. As found in the study, the coping responses that households apply are likely to have cumulative impacts on the household's livelihood. At first glance, some households may appear to be coping with the impacts, but they may be doing so in an unsustainable way. Other authors (Barnett & Whiteside, 2002; Rugalema, 2000) have questioned the use of 'coping' as a concept in a situation where households are constantly struggling to survive, leaving little or no room to respond to livelihood pressures. In this study it was found in that households that are already on the margins of survival can only respond to HIV/AIDS-impacts at the expense of their resilience to other future shocks, which increases their vulnerability to poverty. More resource-endowed households may cope because they are able to mitigate the negative effects of HIV/AIDS on household resources such as labour, for example by using hired labour to compensate for labour lost due to illness. However, in the study area only few HIV/AIDS-affected households managed to do so.

Although non-affected households may experience shocks similar to those who are HIV/AIDS-affected, the latter are more severely affected due to the unique nature of the pandemic. Consistent with the findings of Baylies (2002) HIV/AIDS was found to be a shock with very specific characteristics that undermine individual and communal efforts to secure income generation by mainly affecting the most productive segment of the population. Furthermore, the impacts were found to be clustered (Barnett & Whiteside, 2002). Cases 5.1, 5.2, 5.5 and 5.7 show that the clustering of illness and the loss of young adults pushes households into a downward spiral from which recovery is difficult and which leaves children without means to make their livelihoods. As shown by most case studies involved in the study HIV/AIDS-impacts are gendered in many ways; women are more than men affected in terms of consequences and in terms of susceptibility to HIV-infection.

Chapter 6

Interpersonal social relations: the limits of kinship and friendship – *No (wo)man is an island*[5]

In this study social capital is conceptualized at two levels. Firstly, at the interpersonal level referring to social relations that people have with family, friends and neighbours and whether people believe that they can trust others and others trust them. Secondly, at the community level, referring to membership in community groups, the trust invested in these groups, and the common norms and values held by people. This chapter examines the importance of social capital at the first level specifically for management of HIV/AIDS-impacts and other crises that affect households. Social networks based on kinship and neighbourhoods are an important resource for households. It is assumed that the extended family and the community at large will assist households socially, economically, psychologically and emotionally when they are faced with difficulties. HIV/AIDS-affected households presumably rely on these social assets for help. Yet, as HIV/AIDS continues to strike many households, families and the community at large, it is questionable to what extent these social support networks continue to function as expected. Personal observation, focus group discussions, case studies and the household survey provide the sources for the evidence on this issue presented in this chapter.

6.1 Kinship relations

Social networks are vital to individuals and households in achieving secure livelihoods. Extended families are often assumed to provide their members with assistance, social security and, sometimes, support in economic activities. Family interactions encourage reciprocity and exchange among relatives. The material and emotional support shared freely between family members entails an implicit willingness to return such support. Family relations are also important in fostering trust. Because kinship involves moral obligations it plays a role in care-giving both within households and beyond. In the wake of HIV/AIDS and economic hardship, kinship networks are assumed to provide care for the AIDS-patients and surviving members. However, HIV/AIDS puts a strain on kinship relations in ways that prevent family members to offer support to each other.

While kinship support forms an important source of support, the extent and the nature of kin support vary according to the economic position of the kinship members

[5] Adapted from John Donne, 1572-1631.

and the resources at their disposal. From informal interviews and focus groups discussions (FGD 6 and 7, see Table 3.2) it became evident that assistance from kin is nowadays very minimal as compared to the past. As an old man said:

> *'It is not that the sense of brotherhood is dying but the big problem is poor living and economic conditions for many of the families. Life has become very difficult. Even if your relative is sick, you are unable to assist because of the lack of income.'*

This statement shows that despite the importance of kinship, economic constraints make it difficult to maintain relations with the kin. Resource constraints force people to focus only on their immediate families. In the past, food used to be shared among relatives, but as one of the village leaders explained, this is no longer the case:

> *'You know that long ago we used to get plenty of food, but these days, there is harvest decline, we only harvest small amounts of food, which can hardly satisfy one's own family. Thus, the available food is not sufficient. Despite your concern for your relative, it is difficult to offer food assistance.'*

Households in problems turn to their immediate family members, as Mzee Hogogo, a retired Kilombero Sugar Company officer, explains:

> *'Real relatives were there in the past. Nowadays there is no one who can even pay you a visit, very few do that. Your own children are now your relatives.'*

Mzee Hogogo knows what he is talking about because when his son was hospitalized for a long time he did not get any help from his relatives. They did not provide support when it was most needed, although they did make financial contributions for the funeral. While qualitative methods suggest that there is only reduced and limited kinship assistance, the information collected from the survey shows that relatives are still an important source of support (Table 6.1).

According to the figures in Table 6.1, 58.3 percent of the respondents were able to get financial assistance from their relatives when they were in financial troubles and 42.1 and 45.5 percent, respectively, who were able to get food and medical assistance from relatives. This would indicate that relatives are still an important source of support. However, the data from the focus group discussions and case studies tell a different story, revealing that there is reduced and limited kinship assistance and few people actually manage to secure support from their relatives. The reason for this discrepancy could be that in the survey interviews people tended to respond

Table 6.1. Sources of support for various needs (N=180).

Kind of support	Source of support in %					
	None	Friends and neighbours	Relatives	Religious groups	Employer	Total
Financial	13.3	25.5	58.3	1.2	1.7	100
Food	23.3	33.4	42.1	0.6	0.6	100
Labour	68.3	12.3	19.4	0.0	0.0	100
Job/market opportunity	84.4	11.1	4.5	0.0	0.0	100
Medical help	27.2	26.1	45.5	0.6	0.6	100
Advise	3.3	48.9	40.0	7.8	0.0	100
Emotional	3.9	49.4	28.4	18.3	0.0	100

Source: Household Survey, 2005.

along normative lines rather than relating actual experience. When checking the results of the preliminary analysis of the survey data on this issue, participants in FGD 10 and 11 (see Table 3.2) expressed surprise at the high proportions of reported support by relatives and questioned the truthfulness of the answers.

Although the general opinion is relatives should provide support, a reduced reliance on kinship support can be observed in the qualitative data. A participant of FGD 6 (see Table 3.2) said:

> *'What is noted here is that people have become more self-centred, in such a way that helping somebody is like a burden and that support to others could erode your resources. Others say they have developed European culture – not helping others except for immediate family members. We are now living an urban life.'*

The above statement shows people's perception that kinship has come under the influence of forces that have not only transformed society's orientation but in some ways also affect the functioning of the social system. According to Ottosson (1999) the processes of socio-economic change, urbanization, adoption of Western values, and economic hardship have disrupted family life in Africa. Patterns of family formation and family life continue to undergo considerable change. Modernization and rural-urban dynamics have made it difficult for people to fulfill the socio-economic responsibilities of the extended-family system. Among the dominant factors causing the change in kinship support has been the change in families' economic and material circumstances. As people face difficulties in maintaining kinship ties, they tend to care for their immediate family only. Some studies (Bradley & Weisner, 1997; Caldwell, 1997) suggest that the evidence of the decline of family values is balanced by evidence of continued strength and resilience. Norms of reciprocity and solidarity among kin and life-time connectedness with parents are allegedly still strong. Bradley & Weisner (1997) argue that in Kenya family structures are becoming diverse and changing in form but not in underlying values. They maintain that some functions related to support and care for children and elderly are as strong as ever, though changing in form. However, this is contestable, and this study demonstrates the dramatic effects brought about by different critical forces, including HIV/AIDS, when households need support but find that such assistance is not available.

The following case demonstrates how a person may not have someone to rely on in times of need in spite of having social relationships. The case also illustrates how kinship assistance is constrained in case of prolonged illness.

Figure 6.1 depicts the relationship and social interactions between Mama Dorothy and members of her social network which she considers most important for her.

Kin availability, co-residence and geographical proximity of the available kin influence the support one can get. Figure 6.2 shows a number of persons in Mama Dorothy's kinship network who may be called upon for assistance.

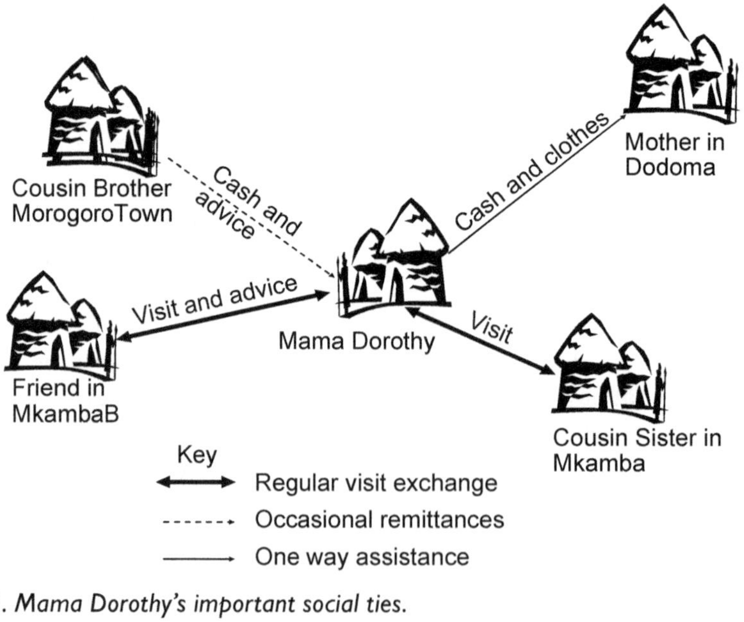

Figure 6.1. Mama Dorothy's important social ties.

Case 6.1. Mama Dorothy: HIV/AIDS-affected, lack of family support.

Mama Dorothy is a divorced woman of sixty-five, with three grown-up children. She belongs to a village court elder's board. She has a vegetable garden near her house. She is from Dodoma but moved to Mkamba in 1975. Her brother back home is the one who looks after their mother. In 1998 Mama Dorothy was able to buy a plot and build the house where the family is currently living. She lives with two of her daughters and two grandchildren who are going to primary school. Her son works in Arusha. Her oldest daughter (42) divorced and came to Mkamba in 1994. She was living alone in the village but moved into her mother's house when she got sick. Two years ago she got herpes zos-ter (skin infection) and has since been frequently ill. Her mother says she has chronic typhoid. When she gets very ill, Mama Dorothy cannot go to her garden or attend the court sessions in the village. Mama Dorothy says: 'Her eyes and her legs are on me, no one else. This is our role as a parent'.

Her second daughter is always busy selling food to get money for her children, but sometimes she gives money for household expenses. They do not get help from the son who lives in Arusha. Mama Dorothy's brother lives in Tabora. They have not been in touch for a long time. Mama Dorothy said it is not easy to get assistance from family members and friends in this situation, because they don't know how long it will take: 'She has been sick for more than a year. Who is going to assist you for a whole year?' Mama Dorothy's cousin who lives in Morogoro town used to send her money, but does not do so anymore, and she does not want to make constant demands on him. Sometimes their neighbours and people from their church group visit them but do not give them any money. Mama Dorothy said that if her daughter were well, she could get a loan and run a business, because she is very good at that. In the present situation people cannot lend her money because they know she is not able to work and the money will be spent on medication. The relatives in Dodoma are also very poor and Mama Dorothy has not been in touch with them. She sold tables and chairs to get money for food and medicine.

When her daughter gets very sick, Mama Dorothy calls in a nurse who lives nearby to come and attend to her at home. She has to pay for the service, but this kind of arrangement costs less than if she were taken to the hospital. Mama Dorothy thinks that her daughter has been bewitched because she was doing very well in her brewing busi-ness. She herself was once taken for shaving after her neighbour accused her of being a witch. She says they were just jealous because as a woman she managed to build a house.

Mama Dorothy's case shows that despite having a considerable number of relatives who represent potential sources of assistance (Figure 6.2), she has not been receiving any substantial assistance from them. Apart from general social interaction with

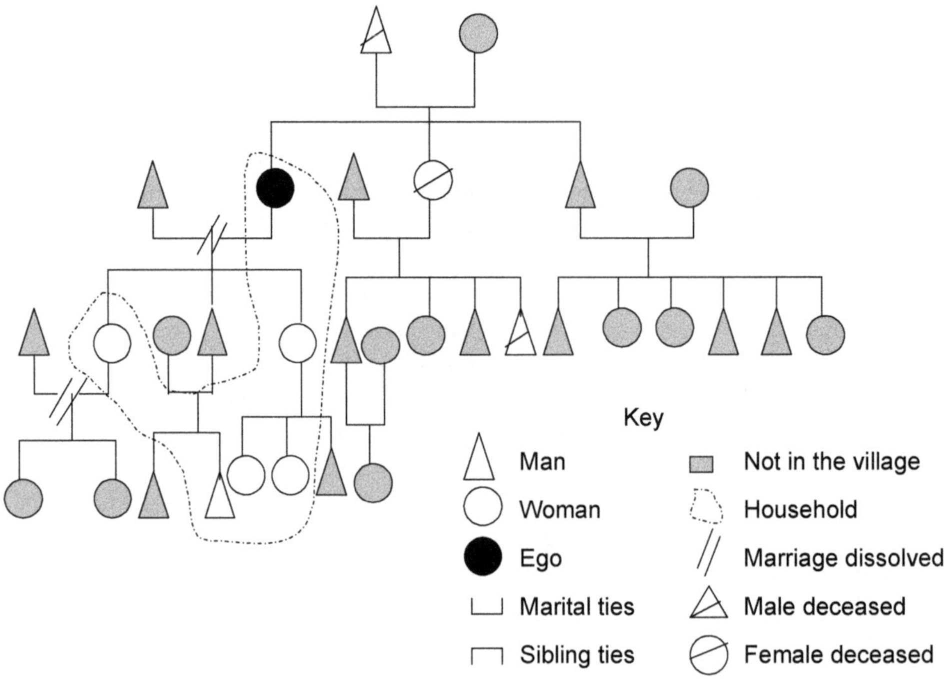

Figure 6.2. Genealogy of Mama Dorothy.

others in the village, such as casual greeting and attending a neighbour's funeral, Mama Dorothy has very few social ties that she considers to be important (Figure 6.1). Proximity is important for practical help, but even a relative and a friend who are living in the same village do not offer any practical or material assistance. They only pay visits and offer emotional support. Mama Dorothy needs help with looking after her sick daughter so that she can earn some money, but she has no one to help her. She also tries to support her mother. Traditionally, the husband's family ought to provide support, but Mama Dorothy is not getting any because she is divorced and lives far away from her husband's family.

Inability to reciprocate and prolonged need for assistance are likely to discourage others from helping relatives with problems. Because of HIV/AIDS impacts, affected households in most cases are left with few resources which make reciprocating in tangible terms difficult. Gillies (1998) says that when a certain point of economic crisis or hardship is reached, reciprocity between households break down. This seems to be the case in Mkamba. Inability to reciprocate makes households in crisis being excluded from informal support mechanisms. On the other hand, affected households may avoid requesting the support they need for fear of overburdening the relationship.

The role of non-resident family members

The social and economic importance of kinship is not always visible when family members are living together. The importance of kinship is also shown among relatives who do not live together but still emotionally and economically depend on one another. Members of the extended family are sources of potential support. Cash remittances by family members indicate the existence of social networks that extend beyond face-to-face interactions (Rose, 1997). In the survey, 43 percent of the respondents reported receiving remittances from non-resident family members. Most of the remittances go from adult children to elderly parents. Remittances are usually cash (87%) and used for household expenses like buying food, paying school fees and meeting medical expenses. Few respondents (13%) reported getting non-cash remittances such as food, clothes and soap. When people do not send remittances it is commonly explained by unemployment, low income, change in familial obligations, or the marriage of the person involved. Commenting on how familial obligations have changed, one old village man said:

> *'Our children have changed these days, we tried very hard to bring them up hoping that they will care for us at old age, but when they go away they forget us. But anyway, you cannot force someone to send you money, if they do is okay, and if they don't it's still fine; we just have to struggle on our own.'*

Geographical distances affect the possibility of maintaining significant links with relatives. Migration has contributed to the weakening of kinship ties by fragmenting the extended family (see Case 6.1) and remittances from those who have migrated are not guaranteed. With the HIV/AIDS surge, remittances are lost when an infected family member returns to his or her household of origin for care and eventually dies. The return to the parents' place increases the pressure on the limited capacity of their household, thereby shifting the burden to the elderly who are poor and vulnerable. The following case study testifies how illness and death of the young adult the parents have been relying on, leaves them in a desperate situation.

As shown in Case 6.2 for parents whose children have died of AIDS the trauma of the death of their children is accompanied by feelings of desperation as to how to cope with the loss of those who supported them.

Case 6.2. Mzee Manda: HIV/AIDS-affected, loss of remittances.

Mzee Manda is 60 years old and lives with his wife and a girl who is a relative. The couple had four children, one daughter and three sons, who are no longer living with their parents. Mzee Manda's daughter died of AIDS in 2000, which he admitted openly. She was 34 and working as a nurse in Morogoro town. Her parents had been paying for her education from their farming income. They produced and sold rice to get money for her school fees while she was in the nursing college. She started getting frequent illnesses two years before she passed away. Back in Morogoro, she could no longer support herself; her parents went and picked her up.

At home, her mother spent a lot of time nursing her daughter who was bedridden for six months before she passed away. It was a very difficult period for the family. Mzee Manda said they had hopes that after educating her she would be able to help her ageing parents. When she was alive, she used to send them money for household expenditures but now they cannot get such assistance. They have to work on their farm to get food and sell some of the pro-duce to get money. At their age they are no longer able to produce much. They rarely get support from their sons in Dar es Salaam.

6.2 Friends and neighbours

Neighbours and friends are another source of support to individuals and households in times of crises. Since most of the households are not originally from Mkamba and have relatives living elsewhere, neighbours and friends become important for immediate help. People had mixed views on the helpfulness of neighbours and friends. Despite the fact that poverty was a problem for the majority of the people in the village, some respondents reported incidences where households in need were assisted with food and money as gifts from friends and neighbours. Borrowing and lending money for medical expenses and other problems is another way of providing assistance among friends and neighbours. Some villagers held negative views on assistance by friends and neighbours, seeing it as not functioning the way it once did and stating that now many people keep to themselves and do not bother about what is happening next door.

Reciprocity is a crucial factor in building and maintaining friendship. Neighbours and friends are motivated to help others hoping that they are helped in return when the need arises. Deducing from the qualitative data it became evident that people who do not want to know about other people's problems are unlikely to be assisted when faced with problems themselves. Funeral ceremonies, however, are truly social events in which many people participate and extensive use is made of social claims.

There are several types of help that friends and neighbours extend to one another. Women were found to help each other in case of problems or festivals based on ties of friendship. There are small groups of five to ten women who are friends and trust each other. They have set a fixed amount of money each member has to contribute for different occasions. For example, for weddings and first Holy Communion each member contributes TShs. 500, one kilogram of rice, and the group give a member concerned a pair of *kitenge*[6]. In the event of the death in a member's household, each member contributes TShs. 200 and as a group they buy bars of soap and a pair of *kitenge*. In case of sickness, they contribute TShs. 200 each only if a member or her immediate family member is hospitalized. The contribution is only given once, and cannot be donated to same household again. Support offered among these women is widespread after the harvesting season, when most of the women are back from their distant farms and have paddy to sell. The same group of friends may engage in an *upatu*[7] scheme. From Focus Group Discussions 7 (see Table 3.2) it appears that one-to-one exchanges among neighbours are not very common due to factors such as lack of trust and lack of resources. While in the past households hosting a festival invited all the members of the community, now in many cases the family concerned will ask people to contribute prior to the ceremony and invites only those who have contributed. The practice works on the principle of balanced reciprocity: a person's contribution to other people's celebrations determines how much the latter will offer in return in the future. It was found that people are more willing to contribute for festivals, where they get something in return, than for problems such as lack of school fees, sickness or food insecurity.

From the household survey results (Table 6.1) it appears that the most common support one gets from neighbours and friends is advice (48.9%) and emotional support (49.4%). For a household that needs material and practical support in a stressed situation but such support is not readily available. One of the women during the focus group discussion said:

> *'Who is there to give you food and money these days? Everyone has to strive for her or his own family (Kila mtu anakufa kivyake).'*

Another woman commented on the matter by saying that:

---

[6] *Kitenge* (*vitenge*-plural) is a piece of cloth that is decorated with a variety of colours and patterns; it is often worn by women around the chest or waist, over the head as a headscarf or as a baby-sling.

[7] *Upatu* is informal group savings whereby participants make regular contributions to a common fund which is given in whole or in part to each contributor in turn.

> *'Even if you have friends, it is just 'on the mouth' (ni kwa mdomo tu). We cannot help each other because our circumstances are the same; if it is business's bad performance then it is likely they experience the same. If it was bad weather, then we are all likely to be affected. Now who is to help the other?'*

Because of widespread poverty in the village families are often too burdened with their own problems to be of much help to others. Some periods of the year are worse than others for getting assistance. For instance, it was reported in the Focus Group Discussion 2 (see Table 3.2) that during the rainy season, known as *masika*, when people are fully engaged in farming activities, most of the households experience food insecurity and low income and it is not easy to get or give support. For Mkamba village, the term *masika* connotes hardship. In their study in South Africa, Carter & Maluccio (2003) also found that the capacity to cope is weakened in communities that suffer covariant shocks that overwhelm the social coping mechanisms in the area.

In the past people worked in each other's field in turns and women looked after each other's children. Households without food borrowed from those who had, while those facing short-term cash crises borrowed from relatives, neigbours and friends. Those from whom assistance was sought were not necessarily better-off in material terms than those who seeking it. What was important was the willingness of people to assist each other and the expectation that when in need of assistance one will get it. But the situation has changed, as a village man says:

> *'It has become exceptional for people to make local brew and invite people to come over and work in their field, this is an old-fashioned activity. Nowadays if you have no money to hire people to work in your plot you are finished.'*

A focus group discussion participant (FGD 1, see Table 3.2) describes the role of money and how its scarcity undermines mutual support relations, stating that:

> *'You know money is everything these days, if you are sick you need money for treatment, you have no food you need money to buy it, basically everything needs money. Then, how is it possible for a person to give to a neighbor some sugar or maize flour that he or she had bought from the very little money a household has been able to make?'*

The size of one's social network determines how much support one gets or is likely to get. On the social-capital scale described in Chapter 3, about 68 percent of the respondents had moderate informal social capital, meaning that they only have one to four people to whom they can turn for support. It also appeared that the assistance from those persons is very limited and unreliable. More than half of the respondents said nobody asked them for assistance during the previous three months. The reasons given were: firstly, they had nothing to give to others and, secondly, people did not ask them for assistance. For those who helped others, few offered their labour, some gave cash (on average TShs. 3,000) and others offered food (on average 1.5 kilograms). Although this study did not establish an objective level of resources needed in the study area per individual per day, the comparison with the average consumption expenditure per person per month in rural areas of TShs. 8,538 (URT, 2002) signify that the quantities of items and cash the respondents were offered is inadequate for households to survive on. It is also worth mentioning that in some instances people were confident that in spite of not being helped now there would be someone to help in the future.

The following case study illustrates how geographical distance and weak ties among relatives limit social support in times of need, and how neigbours and friend may provide assistance, even though their help is not sufficient.

Children are expected to provide emotional and material support to their parents especially during old age and at difficult times. Mama James expects her children to do so but they do not have a reliable income, so life is difficult for all of them. Although she is aware of her dependency on her children, she berates their assistance as inadequate and is completely dissatisfied. Mama James has a considerable number of relatives who could help her but they are living far away and refrain from giving support. Presumably because of her sickness, her husband abandoned her and the children. Since Mama James cannot work anymore to provide for her family herself, the children are deprived of basic necessities such as food and education.

HIV/AIDS influences relationships with neighbours and friends. Since continual interaction is based on give and take, HIV/AIDS-affected and other poor households are unlikely to be able to maintain this exchange. Mama James's neighbour seems to be tired of helping, which she is doing on humanitarian grounds. There are also times she cannot assist her sick neighbour due to lack of food or money. It was even explicitly said by one woman participant during a focus group discussion (FGD 8, see Table 3.2) that: 'No one will be willing to assist someone from January to December knowing that this person will not be able to reciprocate'.

It was found that suspicions of witchcraft make more difficult to access the support that might otherwise be provided by friends and neighbours. People try to minimize contacts with their neigbours to avoid witchcraft allegations. Additionally, stigma

Case 6.3. Mama James: HIV/AIDS-affected, neighbour's assistance, lack of family support.

Mama James, a 45 years-old woman originally from Dodoma, came to Mkamba in 1978. She has four children from two different fathers. Her older daughter (26) who lives in the same village is a widow with two children aged seven and one. Her husband died in May 2004. Mama James's second born is a boy aged 21. He works and lives in the neighbouring village of Ruaha, where he runs a chips kiosk. Mama James's first partner worked as a casual labourer in the sugar cane plantation and left Mkamba in 2002. Mama James's other younger children are a boy and a girl, aged 11 and six years respectively. The boy was supposed to be in grade four but was expelled from school for not having shoes and not paying school contributions. Mama James has been making her livelihood from farming and brewing. She is living with her two young children in a windowless rented room with mud walls and a mud floor, only one small bed and very little furniture. She is living with seven other families in the same house.

Since she started getting ill in July 2004, she has not been able to work. Around the same time the father of her young children left, claiming to go to another village (Mngeta) in the District to look for farming land. He has not been home since. Recently he sent a letter but did not mention anything about coming back. Mama James thinks he has another wife there. Mama James is very weak and has mouth sores, chest pains and a chronic cough. One of her neighbours reported the case to the village health worker, who visited and advised her to take the TB test, but there was no-one to get the equipment from the hospital to take the sample for the test.

She complains that although her daughter lives in the same village, she does not visit her very often. At the time of the interview, the daughter had not shown up for the past five days. The last time she came, she just brought her mother some tea and nothing else, and even the tea was tasteless. Mama James says her elder son regularly brings money for food and other expenses. Her daughter is a food vendor but has stopped the business because the owner claimed back the stall she was using. She is trying to help her mother as much as she can but the problem is lack of money to support both her children and her mother. Mama James knows of her daughter's tight situation but she never stops complaining. There are times when Mama James's daughter does not visit her mother because she has nothing to give her. On other occasions, she buys food on credit from the local shop to cater for her family and her mother's. What-ever she eats is what she takes to her mother. Together with her brother, they buy medicine for her as well. Mama James's neighbours told me that they sometimes force the daughter to sleep in her mother's house to look after her during the night.

Case 6.3. Continued.

Although Mama James lives with other people in the same house, there are only two who help her. They took her to the local dispensary, where she was given painkillers. Mama James does not like going to the local dispensary anymore because they used her money (TShs 1,000) without treating her with medicine. Later, Mama James's neighbour took her to the private dispensary in the village where she was diagnosed with typhoid, malaria and anaemia. Because of a lack of money Mama James could only buy half the dose of medicines prescribed. If they get food, Mama James's young children cook for themselves; if not, their mother tells them to play with other children hoping they will be given food. 'I am just dying of hunger, I am getting weak because I don't have food, otherwise I could have recovered', Mama James says. Another neighbour brought her some maize flour but as she did not have any relish they ended up making porridge without sugar.

Mama James is concerned about how long these good neighbours are going to help her while her own daughter does nothing. Mama James thinks her daughter is greedy, but at the same time might be tired of caring since she has been sick for a long time. Mama James praised one of her neighbours for her regular help. She helps Mama James with almost everything, like carrying water to the bathroom, cooking, and cleaning the room. The caring neighbour said: 'Even though we don't have much, whatever little we have we share with her; she is a human being like us. If I don't have any food, she stays without eating which is bad for her since she is very weak'. She added: 'Even if I don't help her, no one will blame me because she is not my relative and I am not obliged to'.

The local village government mobilized contributions from the village to help Mama James, but the money was not enough to sustain her for more than a few days. The local village leaders feel that they cannot fundraise for her regu-larly, because people should solve their own problems. The people of her ethnic group do not help her. Mama James says: 'It's only by name that I am a member of that tribe, I don't get any help from it'. Mama James has no contact with her relatives back home and cannot think of going back. She fears the blame from her relatives if she falls Ill. She thinks her relatives will blame her, saying 'You spend your life alone and now you are bringing problems to us, one can easily die back home'. She has told her neighbours that if she dies, she would like to be buried in Mkamba and not in her home of origin.

attached to (suspected) AIDS limit the support one can get from neigbours and friends. A lady who had TB was not accepted back into the local brew business. 'No one will buy local beer from me', she says. Such treatment towards the afflicted denies them a chance to forge bonds with people who could be of help. In such circumstances, those who are stigmatized become more vulnerable and have less chance to benefit from social networks.

To examine the relationship between informal social capital (as the dependent variable) and individual and households characteristics (as independent variables) more closely, an ordinal regression analysis was conducted. However, as Table 6.2 shows, the explanatory power of the overall model appears to be limited (14.12 %) and it is not statistically significant ($p=0.1676$). The only two variables in this model that have a significant effect on informal social capital (measured as described in Chapter 3) are effective dependency ratio ($p= 0.077$) and deaths experienced in the household ($p=0.046$). Both are negative relationships, implying that informal social capital is lower with increasing effective dependency ratio and increasing number of deaths in the household. There is no significant effect of age, marital status,

Table 6.2. Factors influencing informal social capital (N=180).

Explanaory variables	B-coefficient	Standard error
Age (years)	-0.0085254	0.0107964
Household headship (1=male)	0.1782449	0.5353644
Education level (1=educated)	-0.2134791	0.3711869
Effective dependency ratio	-0.305654*	0.1730128
Marital status (1=married)	-0.1740269	0.4461121
No. of people with chronic illnesses	-0.1694881	0.2375901
Death/s in the household (1=yes)	-0.6218393**	0.3117801
Estimated household annual income (Tshs)	2.64e-07	2.36e-07
Duration of stay (1= >10 years)	0.3670761	0.4082843
Food security status	-0.0192308	0.0725612
Group membership	0.0490548	0.0297781

LR Chi^2 (10) = 14.12
Prob > Chi^2 = 0.1676
Pseudo R^2 = 0.0261
Log likelihood = -263.05457
*p<0.10, **p<0.05.
Source: Household Survey, 2005.

duration of residence in the village, educational level and number of people with prolonged illness in the household. A non-significant effect of duration of residence may be explained by the fact that most (85%) of the households have been living in the area for more than 10 years. Surprisingly, although membership in groups may result in an increased number of people who trust and help each other, it does not seem to affect informal social capital. Though income and headship are not statistically significant, there was a difference in terms of informal social capital scale between female- and male headed households in the same wealth category. Fewer poor female-headed households (25%) than poor male-headed households (34.5%) have low informal social capital. This could indicate that women are better in mobilizing informal social capital. There are no well-off female- and male-headed households with low informal social capital, which is an indication of a connection between wealth and informal social capital although the indicator income does not score significantly.

From the above, it can be said that the analysis of the survey data offers some clues but yields only a partial picture of what determines people's access to informal social capital and whether it helps them to solve their problems. The qualitative data from the case studies and focus group discussions offers a more holistic picture of the importance of access to and use of informal social capital for households in trouble. In commenting on the limitations of quantitative studies for assessing the economic burden of illness for households Russell (2005:277-278) says that there is scope for case study household research, because it 'can adopt a more naturalistic methodology, seeking to understand the economic burden of illness as it unfolds within the context of a household, and the ways that people in their everyday lives take action to treat illness and cope with its costs.'

6.3 Patron-client relations

Patron-client relationships were found to be another source support in the village although the respondents did not mention it during the survey interview. However, they are also part of social networks and built on norms of reciprocity (though unbalanced) and trust. Patron-client relationships are unequal and in most cases are biased towards patron's vested interests. Different kinds of support can be offered by patrons to their clients. The most popular form of patronage in the village is that between moneylenders and clients. Some support in the form of food may be provided by landowners to persons who work on their land. Another common form of a patron-client relationship is that between shop-keepers and customers.

Moneylenders are very important in the village because of the lack of a regular source of income for the majority of the village population for many months in the year.

Moneylenders are villagers who by different means have managed to accumulate money, from which they can provide loans to others. Some were able to accumulate cash money from the proceeds of their own farming and business activities, others managed to get loans from financial institutions. People take loans for various purposes like farming, medical treatment, and household expenses. Moneylenders have several means, including force and harassment, to ensure repayment. As a rule the interest rates are high.

Usually moneylenders give money to people whom they already know. If not, one has to have a guarantor who will take responsibility in case of defaulting. Moneylenders assess the borrower's socio-economic status, based on borrower's assets base, the ability to produce a good harvest or employment as indicators. They give loans for the amount of money they assume one is able to repay. Past performance of the borrower is also an important criterion. If a person did not repay a former loan the information will circulate among lenders, and the person concerned will not be trusted by other moneylender. Sometimes moneylenders dictate a high interest rate to discourage borrowing, if they are not sure of the borrower's capability to repay. Moneylenders sometimes base their decision on the way the borrower is able to convince them. The criteria used tend to discriminate against very poor households and persons and households that are not able to engage in income-earning activities, such as elderly people and HIV/AIDS-afflicted households.

The period for repayment usually depends on the purpose and the amount of loan taken. If the loan is for other purposes than farming, the repayment period is usually relatively short. Regularly employed people take short-terms loan, which they usually pay back at the end of the month. Loans for family maintenance (medical care and food) can be as low as TShs. 2000, which has to be paid back within a short time, usually after two to four weeks. The money for loan repayment can be obtained from casual work wages, sale of local brew (especially for women) or from any other income-generating activity. As said, failure to pay for may affect one's possibility of getting loans in the future. Farming loans are usually given from December to March, which is the critical time for rice and maize farming. The minimum amount loan for farming activities is TShs. 10,000. Farming loans are usually repaid after harvest, preferably in kind. Most of the people interviewed said that the interest rates charged are very high, but are forced to comply as there are no other means get the money needed. This is illustrated in the following statement by a village woman:

> *'You know poverty is very bad, when faced with a problem you have no where to run to except to moneylenders who may give you money to solve the problem at hand, but what you are paying in return, is far much higher than what you took, but we have no means.'*

Loan servicing seems to increase poverty to the households involved.

There are moneylenders who collect paddy from the debtor's fields even before the harvest is transported home. This is done to make sure that the borrowers do not dodge paying. Many households are trapped into poverty as they are trying to service the loan. There are cases where households ended up repaying with all produce harvested, becoming food insecure as a consequence. If there is no harvest at all, the loan is extended to another farming season with additional interest. In case of pensioners and employees the moneylender keeps their bank pass books, to force them to withdraw the money to repay the loan in the presence of the moneylender.

People also seek loans from moneylenders because they do not require prior financial contributions as is common in the saving-and-credit groups in the area. Other credit schemes require one to be a member with shares, a condition that is difficult for many to fulfill. Problems may come unexpectedly which such groups are not in position to deal with on a short notice. In the past the government revenue authority wanted to ban moneylenders operating in the area, but the villagers insisted that they should not be stopped because it is the only way people can access loans that are not provided by the government and NGOs.

As said, moneylenders charge high interests, but in some instances no interest is paid for short-term loans, depending on the lender-borrower relationship. Despite strict follow-up mechanisms moneylenders interviewed complained of defaulters, because people fail to pay because of bad harvest but also some people just do not want to pay. Only in a few cases this led to legal actions and court intervention, because moneylenders find legal procedures too involving and time-consuming. To show that they also appreciate the ties they have with other people in the village, one of the moneylenders said:

> *'I feel delighted to offer such service in the village because by doing so I have been able to make a number of friends. There are times they even give me more than what they were supposed to repay, so it is not only a matter of money but also of friendship.'*

Another type of patron-client relationship is between shopkeepers and their clients. This is an arrangement whereby people take mainly household items such as food, kerosene, matchboxes and soap from the shops without immediate payment. The payment is done later, though the time is not fixed. There is no interest charged on the items taken. Shopkeepers keep records of every household involved. This arrangement is beneficial to both households and shop owners. Households are able to get their daily basic needs without cash and shopkeepers are assured of customers even though payment comes later. Most of the shop owners are willing to help households in this way because people in the village often do not have the money for cash payments. Based on their knowledge of the people in the village, shopkeepers establish the average total amount the household concerned can shop for. Failure to pay the accumulated debt will bar the household from getting more items from the shop. Such arrangements are wide-spread in the village and facilitate various households to cope with food insecurity when they have no cash, provided that they are able to pay previous debts. Their underlying principle is trust among the people involved.

6.4 Trust at interpersonal level

Mutual relations and exchanges are based on trust, which is built-up as a result of continual interactions. People usually help each other if there is trust between or among them and if one believes that others might help them in future if need be. At face value, relationships in the village seem to be harmonious. The results from the household survey indicate that people get support and assistance from relatives, neighbours and friends, which may imply they are trusted. However, as described above qualitative methods revealed a somewhat different picture. Different from what is often assumed, assistance from extended family, friends and neighbours seems to be rare, inadequate or not available at all. Only 17 percent of the respondents trusted their neighbours and friends to look after their baby or sick relative. The apparent lack of social support in the village can be partly explained by lack of interpersonal trust, which the people themselves attribute to economic hardship, witchcraft accusations, and ethnic diversity.

Lack of interpersonal trust has curtailed social networks and reciprocal relations in the village. When respondents and key informants were asked if villagers trust each other, many involved in the study responded in a negative way. Lack of trust is manifested in various ways. People in the study area said you cannot judge someone from his/her appearance, as people are different; there are those to trust and some are not to be trusted. Where there is no trust and where people are not able to reciprocate, relations with neighbours and friends become strained. Witchcraft suspicions and accusations reflect deteriorating trust among neighbours and friends as stated by a village woman:

> *'Even if I know my neigbours do not have food, I cannot provide them with food for fear of being accused of witchcraft in case a member of that household gets sick, I don't want to be harassed and be taken to the "salon" for shaving.'*

One participant of the focused group discussions (FGD 6, see Table 3.2) said:

> *'I knew that my neighbour has a patient in his house, so I went to visit them twice. When I went for the third time, I was told they have moved the patient from this place to another village. Three days later, that person died, so I was surprised, why they had to cheat me on that. Was it that they thought I am the one responsible for his sickness? I could not even go to the funeral for fear of being attacked.'*

The following account indicates that such fears of being accused of witchcraft are justifiable. During the Focus Group Discussion 6 (see Table 3.2) an account was given of the following incident. A man was shaving his son's hair. The neighbour's son demanded a hair cut as well, so the man shaved him too and explained to his neighbour what had happened. The neighbour was not happy about this and suspected the man of tampering with his son. He took him to a ten-cell leader to discuss the matter and the man was later taken for the 'salon' for shaving (cf. Chapter 4).

Relatives accuse each other of witchcraft. For example, during an in-depth interview Mama Kandoro (Case 6.4) claimed that her son, reportedly to have died of AIDS, was bewitched by her brother. She said it was not normal for a person to be sick for so long unless he was bewitched. Mama Kandoro summoned her brother for the cleansing ritual but her son did not get better and passed away. Even after the cleansing ritual, Mama Kandoro did not request any assistance from her brother although he was in position to help her.

Economic difficulties seem to affect interpersonal trust as well, as a woman in a focus group discussion (FGD 7, see Table 3.2) describes:

> *'I think what causes mistrust is the bad economic situation. Nowadays our incomes are very low, so in many cases one is forced to borrow let's say Tshs 50,000, but when it comes to the repayment, one fails to even pay part of the loan, say 10,000/, for lack of money. In this case it will be difficult to approach the same person for another loan because s/he no longer trusts you. Bad economic conditions make people seen as dishonest.'*

People's economic situation has a bearing on their interaction and capability of material exchanges. As we have seen, there has been a decline in people's incomes due to low farming outputs, low wages and unemployment. Because of their poverty, even people living in one house are suspicious of one another. For instance, in rented houses people have a common cooking place, where each one can easily see what others cook. If it happens that a housemate frequently cooks meat, which is expensive, this person may be suspected of getting the money for it by witchcraft. Allegations like this can be attributed to jealousy of people who cannot make ends meet, leading to feelings of hostility towards people who are better-off that translate into witchcraft accusations.

Ethnic diversity is another factor contributing to the decline of interpersonal trust. People tend not to trust people from other ethnic groups. It was said during a focus group discussion (FGD 7, see Table 3.2) that people interact less frequently with people from other ethnic groups. For example, there are some women *upatu* networks, which did not function because some members from a particular ethnic group isolated themselves from the group, which led to the group's dissolution. Ethnic diversity in a migrant community like Mkamba seems to negatively affect trust and social interaction. People's mobility brings in people who are not rooted in the area and who are unlikely to trust each other.

6.5 Interpersonal relations and gender

As discussed earlier on, there are differences between the social networks of men and women. Studies have shown that women are more likely to be involved in informal exchange relations with relatives and friends than men who tend to rely more on formal relationships (Mayoux, 2001; Silvey & Elmhirst, 2003; Oorschot & Arts, 2004). In the study area more women than men were involved in informal rotating saving funds which in Tanzania are commonly known as *upatu* and are similar to the rotating saving-and-credit schemes (ROSCA) found in other countries in Africa. The system comprises between five to ten women who know and trust each other. They accumulate funds from all involved and at the end of the week or month, depending on the time-frame set by members, the amount accumulated is given to each of the participants in turns. Some give cash and other purchase household items such as mattresses, furniture and others household assets requested by their fellow friend. Many women prefer receiving household items to cash because they are afraid that they will spend the money on meeting urgent needs. Saving groups are more active after the harvesting season when women have the money to contribute to the scheme. Women who are not taking part in such saving groups say that they lack the money to make the daily or weekly contributions.

During the Focus Group Discussion 6 and 7 (see Table 3.2) it was said that the most common men networks in the area are drinking groups comprising men who share a beer in the local bar. If you don't have the money to buy a beer, you can be treated to it but you have to return the favour in the future. In most cases these relationships begin and end at the local bar, although in some cases they evolve into friendship. There are no *upatu* arrangements among men because of lack of mutual trust. There was a feeling among both men and women that *upatu* schemes do not work for men. If there is one the cycle is likely to collapse before all members get their turn because those who have got their money may not contribute for others. As one man in Focus Group Discussion 6 (see Table 3.2) said: 'We men do not trust each other, so is difficult to have a sustainable relationship, and is even more difficult when it involves money'.

Because of their domestic responsibilities, women tend to nurture social relations to reduce risks and cope with the various problems the household may face. Results from Focus Group Discussion 7 (see Table 3.2) indicate that women play a crucial role in cultivating and maintaining interpersonal relations in order to cope with daily problems. As one woman explains:

> *'Even if my husband is around, in case of food shortage or any other problem, I am the one to struggle and look for ways to solve those problems by asking assistance from my neighbours or friends and sometimes even asking for a short-term loan. I can't just sit and watch my children suffering.'*

Moreover, it was noted that in male-headed households, men may be taking advantage of the female household members' networks to solve their problems.

When kind and source of support (Table 6.3) between female- and male-headed households are compared, as done in Table 6.3, it shows that there are some differences, though they are not significant. For all categories except for that of assistance with finding a job, support from friends and neighbours scores higher for female-headed households than male-headed ones.

6.6 Discussion and conclusion

In the absence of widespread formal social security schemes in Tanzania, most households rely on their own resources and assistance from relatives to cope with the effects of AIDS and other predicaments. Beyond the immediate and extended family, households in crisis turn to friends and neighbours for support. Informal social ties that operate in Mkamba village include relatives, neighbours, friends and informal interest groups. There are also patron-client relations between moneylenders or shop owners and their clients that can be a source of support as well.

Extended family ties and kinship relations have always been regarded as an important source of social, economic and practical support, ensuring that the needs of individuals were attended to within the family. Because of the moral obligations involved, kinship networks allegedly function as a resort for social support for their members.

Table 6.3. Sources of support by household headship category (N=180).

Kind of support and household headship		Source of support in %					
		None	Friends and neighbours	Relatives	Religious groups	Employer	
Financial	Male	12.6	25.2	58.7	1.4	2.1	$\chi 2= 4.26$
	Female	16.2	27.0	56.8	0.0	0.0	p=0.51
Food	Male	23.8	32.9	42.0	0.7	0.7	$\chi 2=2.30$
	Female	21.6	35.1	43.2	0.0	0.0	P=0.80
Labour	Male	68.5	11.2	20.3	0.0	0.0	$\chi 2=3.61$
	Female	67.6	16.2	16.2	0.0	0.0	P=0.30
Job/Market	Male	83.2	11.2	4.9	0.0	0.0	$\chi 2=2.28$
opportunity	Female	89.2	8.1	2.9	0.0	0.0	P=0.51
Emotional	Male	4.9	47.6	28.0	19.6	0.0	$\chi 2=6.91$
	Female	0.0	56.7	29.0	13.5	0.0	P=0.14

Source: Household survey, 2005.

Contrary to the assumption that this function is still strong in rural areas (Nkurunziza & Rakodi, 2005), in the study area notable changes in the functioning of traditional extended family support system were found. Due to widespread poverty individuals cannot count on their relatives for help. The trend towards family nuclearization has also limited the support of the extended family to poor and vulnerable family members. While migration enabled household members to earn income elsewhere, it also negatively affected kinship ties. Growing mobility has caused the geographic dispersal of the members of kinships networks, leading to loosened social ties and weakened responsibilities and reciprocity within families. Because of low incomes, relatives are often not able to keep in touch and provide assistance to each other. Even when relatives are living close by, which would allow frequent exchange of care, food and practical support in case of a household member's prolonged illness these were found not to be available. These processes are illustrated by Cases 6.1 and 6.3. When support from siblings is not forthcoming providing care is left to elderly parents, especially women. For women the informal social networks appear to be more important as a source of support than for men. Women need informal networks to cope with different problems in the household and their participation in women's groups enables them to accumulate resources that they otherwise would not have been able to get.

Qualitative information collected shows that money has gained precedence over exchanges in-kind, which were previously important in maintaining mutual relations. In many interactions now cash is the medium of exchange. Money was seen by many involved in the study to be the most important asset, but there are limited opportunities to earn money because of unemployment and low returns from agriculture and non-farm activities. Furthermore, the flows of remittances have diminished. Meanwhile, the cost of living is high and expenses for health services are increasing. As people are unable to earn enough for their families, they have nothing left for others. People are in an increasingly difficult position to ask for and provide support. Increased poverty and deteriorating living conditions among the people seems to have affected mutual help among relatives, friends and neighbours. Similar to what Berry (1993) found because of widespread poverty the ability of household to provide security for one another is weakened. It was found that HIV/AIDS-affected households are struggling to make their living, with no or minimum support from their relatives, friends and neighbours, as those are equally affected. Caution should therefore be taken not to overestimate the role of social networks in enabling households cope with HIV/AIDS impacts and other shocks. The significance of bonding social capital among people with a more or less similar socio-economic status is jeopardized by a widespread crisis because it affects them equally and simultaneously, leaving them all in the same trouble.

Informal support systems, previously effective even in resource-poor environments, are weakening under the strain of dwindling resources. Mobilization of resources within the social network becomes difficult in case of prolonged illnesses and because of HIV/AIDS-related stigma. Moreover, kinship and friendship relations impose obligations to provide assistance to other members based on the principle of reciprocity. When members are no longer able to contribute as expected, they loose their access to the social support provided by the informal networks. HIV/AIDS effects destabilize reciprocity by stripping households off the resources necessary for mutual exchange. As pointed out by Beuchelt *et al.* (2005) mutuality is the main motivation for helping each other, and when not guaranteed or anticipated, support is limited. Similar to the findings of this study Bossart (2003) found that HIV/AIDS-afflicted individuals receive little or no help from their social networks.

In a situation where family members are dispersed over different locations, the relations with friends and neighbours become an important alternative source of social support. However, the findings of this study indicate that people's relations with friends and neighbours cannot be taken for granted. Although unequal in status, patron-client relations are an important form of support in the village. Interpersonal informal social networks have been found to be severely constrained by lack of trust in the community because of the combination of poverty, ethnic diversity, and stigma attached to HIV/AIDS. The proliferation of witchcraft accusations reflects the decline of trust in the study area. Though people claim that the cleansing ritual fosters understanding and harmony among people in the community, discussions with key informants show that even after ritual the relations between accused and accusers are likely to remain strained. Even individuals and households who already have strong informal social networks and are economically better-off find themselves unable to exploit their potential because of widespread witchcraft accusations and ethnic diversity. Lack of trust affects the viability of social networks, necessary for building social capital, one of the assets necessary for helping households cope with problems.

Chapter 7

A community in distress: the role of community-level social capital

This chapter specifically addresses HIV/AIDS impacts at the community level. In this study community social capital is defined by the ability of community members to work collectively towards a common goal through membership in groups and participation in communal activities and the level of trust among members in the community. Community-level social capital was measured by participation in formal groups and communal activities. Because of the interlocking nature of social relations, it is difficult to make a clear-cut distinction between formal and informal social networks. In this study, formal group refers to any group of people registered or not, who get together regularly for a common activity and have agreed upon some rules to guide group operations and performance. While the primary objective of these groups may not be social interaction, their gatherings shape common social norms among members which may build social capital. Participation in group activities and other interpersonal networks may enhances trust among people who may come together to tackle common problems and help vulnerable households. The contexts in which people are living in determine their ability to work for a collective goal. There is a range of inter-related factors as outlined in Chapter 4 that influence households and community process in the study area, which also indicate the complexity and context specificity of social capital and HIV/AIDS impacts. Although there are some opportunities to improve livelihoods, as evidenced by falling incomes in Mkamba poverty is deepening, which intensifies people's vulnerability and exclusion of some groups. These problems not only put strains on households' responses to shocks and crises but also hamper the community to work towards a common goal. This chapter elucidates the importance of contextual specificity in assessing impacts of HIV/AIDS epidemic and also shows that the community context is a key feature in understanding how social capital is generated and maintained, drawing on qualitative village-level data as well as quantitative household-level data.

7.1 Social groups and organizations: inclusion and exclusion

At the community level, local groups are the manifestation of social capital. Formal groups include social ties that exist within the context of a formal organization and these groups have elements like bylaws, regular meetings, and minutes. The members of these groups not necessarily belong to each other's immediate circle of close contacts that informal social capital is made up of. These organizations may represent safety-nets for the members in times of crises, but not for non-members.

There is an increase of people's membership in formal groups for the past five years as reported by 73.5 percent of the respondents. From the group inventory it was found that in 1984 there was one group and since then the number of groups has increased. For example, there were six new groups formed in 2004 alone. This is probably because as people's economic condition becomes difficult they come together to solve household and community day-to-day problems to improve their situation. It could also be as a result of the role of NGOs. An individual's decision to participate in groups is linked to the potential benefits that can be derived from it. The majority of the respondents (78.4%) joined the groups for security in case of problems such as illness and death. Twenty percent said they joined groups to improve their household livelihoods by accessing resources and services that they would not get on their own. Few respondents (1.6%) said they joined for a sense of belonging and emotional and spiritual support.

7.1.1 Formal groups in the study area

i. Sugarcane out-growers and saving and credit groups

The most prominent formal production group in the village is that of sugarcane out-growers, which is among the village groups forming the KCGA (Kilombero Cane Growers Association). The group comprises men and women who are sugarcane out-growers. Most sugarcane out-growers are obliged to become members of the group, since the Sugarcane Company does not deal with individual farmers. Members benefit from extension services, assistance with sugarcane harvest, transportation as well as credits to invest in their sugarcane plots. The group deal with issues related to sugarcane production, and does not serve any other purposes like assisting members in solving problems of everyday care and subsistence. As a rule, membership to this group requires an entrance fee and contributions that poor farmers are not able to pay. There is an entrance fee (TShs. 1,000) and an annual contribution (TShs. 10,000). Different from other groups, a member must own a sugarcane plot on a minimum of one acre. As shown in Figure 4.3 in Chapter 4, every member of the village sugarcane production groups is automatically a member of KCGA for which s/he has to pay TShs. 3,000 as a membership fee. Many people in the village are not able to engage in sugarcane farming because it is a capital-intensive crop, and many have no plots near the factory due to land shortage in the village.

Although some of the sugarcane out-growers get loans from the National Microfinance Bank (NMB), most of them get loans from the Udzungwa Saving and Credit Cooperative (SACCO). The cooperative is formally registered under the Cooperative Society Act of 1991. It has 1,665 members, 400 of which are women. Any person from Kidatu

Division[8] can become a member of this group provided s/he pays an entrance fee TShs. 5,000, and buy at least ten shares worth TShs. 10,000 each. Members get dividends after three years from accumulated yearly dividends. The cooperative started collaboration with CRDB[9] in 2002, which gave them capital money to provide loans to interested people. According to one cooperative official, the cooperative provides easy loans that do not require an applicant to follow lengthy bureaucratic procedures associated with formal banks and other financial institutions. Although loan application procedures are easier than in formal financial institutions, non-member key informants expressed their concern on securing loans from this group, if one is not a sugarcane out-grower. They felt that the conditions for becoming a member favour the well-to-do households and not the poor. For other business loans, the conditions and procedures are too complicated for poor household to meet. It requires one to have a business stall with on-going activities and also to get reference and affirmation papers from various government institutions in the village. This process seems to be lengthy and time consuming for many poor households. Hence, many people are not able to apply for loans. Both the sugarcane out-growers groups and the saving-and-credit group are mainly ways to organize sugarcane out-growers and provide them with access to financial capital.

Since many people are not aware of their HIV status and even if they are do not disclose it, it is likely that there are SACCO members who are affected. However, data from the household survey shows that there is only one identified HIV/AIDS-affected household involved in this group. This may suggest that there could be few HIV/AIDS-affected members in the saving-and-credit group. According to Murray (2005) membership in saving and credit groups is generally most useful to households before the impact of AIDS becomes severe, when people are still well enough to save money and to use loans for productive activities. The majority of HIV/AIDS-affected households identified in the study were found to be too poor to become members of saving-and-credit groups, because they cannot afford the relatively high initial financial contribution.

ii. Women groups

Women groups create an opportunity for women to meet and work together to improve their personal and household well-being. The groups that discussed here differ from those discussed in Chapter 6 because, although not legally registered they

[8] The third lower level in the Tanzanian government administrative structure

[9] Cooperative Rural Development Bank which offers microfinance services to intermediary microfinance institutions such as community banks, SACCOS, and financial NGOs which in turn provide financial services to their individual customers.

do have rules and bylaws governing membership and their operations. The groups are usually small with membership ranging from ten to fifty women. The groups have limited organizational and financial capacity. They do not have links with other groups outside the village and their income is raised from within the group. Though there are fourteen groups, there are also reports of lack of capital to run the group, misunderstandings, and poor leadership that cause groups to dissolve. All except one of the fourteen groups have no common projects because of management problems. Generally, the groups aim at helping members in case of problems such as illness and death of immediate family members as well as during festivals. The contributions by members are higher than those in the groups described in Chapter 6. Each member has to contribute Tshs.200 in case of illness and Tshs 200 to 500 in case of death if the death has occurred in the village. If the death did occur in the village, the groups contribute Tshs.10,000 on average to the household concerned. In case of a death the members also are expected to contribute labour and food. As I observed, many groups have 'uniforms', such as usually identical T-shirts and *kitenge* or *khanga*[10], that they wear at funerals or festivals.

Some women groups are involved in beer-brewing, though the women work individually. These are political (UWT[11]) women groups that are aligned to the ruling party (CCM). Though they operate under the umbrella of UWT, they are not involved in its political agenda. By specific arrangements they are allowed to use the UWT bars in the village to sell their beer and generate income. Membership is only for women who are CCM members. In turns, individual women make the local brew and other members of the group help with selling it. Other women groups were formed as a condition for participation in NGO activities. After the group is formed, the members receive training on entrepreneurship and business management, are checked for their loan eligibility, and are finally given loans to invest in individual projects.

Though the women groups were established through friendship ties to assist each other in case of problems and run their businesses, some of them have incorporated *upatu* activities, which are better organized than the *upatu* arrangements of friends and neighbours discussed in Chapter 6. They are larger, have written bylaws, regular meetings and keep records. After everyone has had their turn in receiving the contributions, they may choose to continue and start another cycle or may stop. The frequency of contributions ranges from daily, to weekly or even monthly. Weekly

[10] It is the same as *kitenge* (See Chapter 6) but relatively smaller in size.

[11] Stands for Umoja wa Wanawake wa Tanzania- (Tanzania Women Union) and aims at uniting women through groups at different administrative levels. At first these groups had to run economic activities, but these failed due to financial mismanagement. Currently, they are just a political organization, which inspires women to undertake activities together.

contributions are most common. The total amount of money that can be given to a member ranges from TShs. 10,000 to 100,000. Groups with many members can split into smaller groups with shorter cycles. Long cycles tend to discourage people from participating. According to women key informants regular contributions to a formal *upatu* are only possible for women with a steady income. This excludes very poor women. As one woman told me:

> *'I am making rice buns everyday, out of it I get about TShs. 500 to 1,000 profit, depending on how good the day is. On average my daily food expenses are about TShs. 1,500, so the profit I make cannot even feed my family. I know the upatu arrangement is good but where will I get money for weekly contributions. Getting money for daily food is a problem, how will it be possible to get the money for the group's contribution?'*

The *upatu* schemes are built on trust among their participants, who know each other and who may either come from the same location or share common characteristics or engage in a common activity. For the groups which are formed for *upatu* only, members are carefully recruited, because in case of default there are no legal means to solve the matter. Recruitment relies on the reputation of a person. Though membership recruitment is done with great care, there is always the risk of defaulting members as a result of declining income, the death of a member and dishonesty. *Upatu* schemes are popular among women because they involve few transaction costs and because of their predictability, since one's turn to get the money is known in advance. They also give members access to a relatively large amount of money that would otherwise be difficult to accumulate.

iii. Burial groups

These groups consist of either a few households or individuals belonging to the same ethnic group or living in the same neighbourhood. Members contribute both services and money to the group, in turn for which the group provides assistance to members in the event of death. The groups run according to the rules agreed upon by members and are open to people from different background (though some are along ethnic lines) who are willing to adhere to group rules and conditions. Inability to adhere to group rules may lead to expulsion. People formed burial groups because they realize that, by themselves, they would be unable to meet the funeral expenses or the expenses of transporting the body to their place of origin. Bereaved families get more than financial support: they also receive emotional support, help with transport and preparation of food, and in-kind donations. There are different in-kind and cash contributions by members at such occasions. Burial groups work in different ways. There are groups that spontaneously contribute at the time of death, while in other groups people make contributions over a period of time and funds are made available to the bereaved families at the time of the funeral. Such groups give on average TShs. 20,000 in case of death of an immediate family member. Members also offer their labour in performing various activities during funerals. The groups differ from ROSCAs in that the funds are not given on rotation but are allocated to households at the time of death. Some burial groups have assets such as furniture, cooking pots, and other utensils needed for feasts and funerals which a member can use free of charge. Non-members may hire them, which generates money for the group.

People from the same ethnic group have formed burial groups, which are important because they allow members to be buried in their place of origin. There is an entrance fee, monthly contributions, and also have by-laws to keep the group running. Monthly contributions differ from one group to the other. It ranges between TShs. 200 and Tshs 500 per household. The group usually assists the family to transport the body home and finance funeral activities. It also contributes to burials that take place in the village if that is the family's wish. These services can only be given to members of a particular ethnic group who are registered as member of the burial group and fulfill their membership obligations.

iv. Religious groups

Participation in religious groups was reported to be important for a sense of identity and belonging. Within the major religious groups, there are other groups of people formed for diverse purposes. Roman Catholics have smaller groups consisting of a number of households who pray together and provide spiritual guidance to each other. The groups do not provide specific material assistance to their members. However, it was found that occasionally the Church can offer assistance to the poor and the needy ones. There is one Lutheran Women group that provides support to orphans and widows of their Church only. There are also two main Muslim groups in the village, comprising Shi'a and Sunni muslims respectively, who mostly offer moral and spiritual assistance to their members.

7.1.2 Bridging social capital

Contacts with other groups create an opportunity to interact with others and access external resources. Close ties are necessary to help group members cope on a day-to-day basis, but these ties sometimes may not be very useful in helping the members to get out of their hardships (cf. Putnam, 2000). Most of the groups identified operate in just one village and have no links with other groups inside and outside the village. The lack of connections with other groups is perhaps due to the fact that they are not yet well established and have limited resources. The groups enable members 'get by' but lack the connections (bridging social capital) that could help them 'getting ahead'. While high-level intra-group cohesion is positive, lack of inter-group linkages is problematic for a poor community like Mkamba village, because it constrains access to information and financial resources of other social groups, including those outside the village. It was evident from the interviews with group leaders interviewed that their groups cannot deal with the members' problems once the group's local resources and capacities are exhausted.

7.1.3 Non-governmental organizations

Non-governmental organizations form an important part of civil society. In Mkamba there are few NGOs operating in the community. Although not based on membership, they bring local people together for activities benefiting the community. Through continuous interaction strong bonds may be formed and trust built among those involved. Non-Governmental Organization in the area includes MAI (Mazingira Institute of Tanzania), a locally-based NGO that is active in poverty alleviation and public health, including raising HIV/AIDS awareness, facilitating youth groups and environmental conservation initiatives. AFREDA, an organization based in Dar es Salaam, runs its activities in Mkamba by targeting women entrepreneurs who run a diversity of businesses. It offers business training and provides loans to women only. Women are mobilized to form groups, and these groups act as a guarantee to each woman taking a loan. Women participating in AFREDA groups are encouraged to take up income-generating activities such as food vending, small-scale trade and handicrafts.

Specifically for HIV/AIDS-related activities, there is a national organization called SHDEPHA^{+} (Service Health and Development for People living positively with HIV/AIDS). Its Kilombero branch is located in the neighbouring village Ruaha and was established to help people living with HIV/AIDS. Members are recruited from the whole Kilombero district. The organization deals with counseling and testing, home-based care, provision of ARVs and prevention activities (mainly by distributing condoms). Members pay TShs. 3,000 and TShs. 1,000 as entrance fee and annual contribution, respectively. When I visited the organization's offices, 187 people had volunteered for the HIV/AIDS test, 20 people were found positive and there were 9 people who were on anti-retroviral drugs. The organization has not attracted many members. According to the organization's secretary, people do not like to be associated with it because then it would be known that they are HIV/AIDS-infected, which would invite stigmatization. According to the same official there were no members from Mkamba village. Apart from the reason mentioned above this may also be due to lack of money to pay the fees or not being aware of the organization's existence.

7.2 Participation in groups

Most groups have specific rules for membership and benefits. Members have to pay entrance fees, annual contributions and must comply with conditions as stipulated in bylaws, like regularly attending meetings. Order and discipline are maintained by imposing fines for various offences such as late arrival and missing the meetings without notification. Failure to adhere to group rules leads to expulsion. These groups are governed by the principle that all members should benefit equally from the group. In most cases membership is for individuals, only one group has households as members. This is a neighbourhood group made up of different households that help each other in case of illness and death. Men from these households make financial contributions and women take part in activities such as visiting the sick and cooking during funerals.

In the survey respondents were asked about group membership of themselves or any other household member. Over 45 percent of the households involved in the survey indicated to have one member or more in one or more groups. On average each member was a member of 1.3 groups (range from one and six groups). The majority (74%) is a member of just one group. Financial constraints are the main factor that limits membership in multiple groups. All groups except two are not formally registered. Two groups have been registered under the Cooperative Act of 1991. Membership size is crucial for effective performance of a group. It ranges from 13 to 215. Attendance is an indicator of participation. About 70 percent of group members attended one meeting per month, which is the obligatory for most groups. Only 10 percent of the members did not attend for lack of time being engaged in income-generating activities. Membership fees – paid either monthly or annually – range from TShs. 100 to 100,000.

Determinants of group membership

Personal and households characteristics such as gender, age, health status, household size and economic status influence membership in groups. Table 7.1 presents the findings of the binary logistic regression on determinants of group membership.

Table 7.1 shows that age of the member, duration of stay in the village, household income, and being moderately food insecure are statistically significant. This suggests that the likelihood of being a member of a group increases with age (the survey results show that there were few members in their twenties) and household income.

Table 7.1. Group membership determinants (N=180).

Explanatory variables	B-coefficient	Standard error
Constant	-3.538	1.317
Age of member (years)	0.035**	0.014
Gender of member (1=male)	-0.414	0.431
Member's education level (1=educated)	-0.126	0.431
Gender household head (1=male)	0.089	0.521
Household size	0.076	0.079
No of people with chronic illnesses	-0.184	0.298
Duration of stay in the village (1=>10 years)	0.040**	0.020
Estimated household annual income (Tshs)	0.000***	0.000
Food security status		
Food secure (*Reference*)		
Food insecure	-0.118	0.489
Moderately food insecure	0.853*	0.464

Dependent variable =Group membership (1=yes, 0 = no)
-2 Log likelihood = 215.432
Cases predicted correctly 77.5 percent
*p<0.10, **p<0.05 and ***p<0.01.
Source: Household Survey, 2005.

As expected, duration of stay in the village is positively and significantly associated with group membership. More than two-thirds of group members interviewed have lived in the area for more than ten years. Longer duration of stay in an area provides the opportunity for building social capital through interactions that enable people to develop strong ties and dense networks and to engage in reciprocal relations. Food security is partly related to membership in groups. Households that are moderately food insecure seem to engage in groups more often than food insecure and food secure households. During the Focus Group Discussion 5 (see Table 3.2), it was reported that those who are poor do not have the time and money to donate to groups. Moderately food-insecure households are likely to have relatively more time and money to contribute to groups. Their engagement in groups offers a way of protection against future food shortages and a means to mobilize resources for their livelihoods.

Household size, household headship, educational level and the number of people with chronic illness in the household do not have a significant effect on group membership. Although the number of people with chronic illness in the household does not show any statistical significance, the relationship is negative. This indicates that as the number of household members with chronic illnesses increases, the likelihood of becoming a member of a group decreases. That households with members with prolonged illnesses are not likely to take part in community groups is demonstrated by Case 7.2 below. As Case 7.1 shows, for a household that is not affected by prolonged illness and is relatively well-off, the situation is different. The two cases show how health and economic status influence group membership.

Poor households have problems making ends meet, leaving little to invest in groups. Becoming HIV/AIDS-affected aggravates the situation, as the following case study shows.

The cases above demonstrate higher returns of social capital for the wealthy and greater barriers to participation for the poor. They also show the importance of good health and availability of cash, which are also essential for participation in groups. Non-poor, food-secure households seem to be able to diversify their memberships

Case 7.1. Mama Maiko: well-off household, group membership.

Mama Maiko is married with two children. Though she did not complete primary education, she has become a successful business woman in the village. She owns a restaurant near the central market in the village. She makes cakes, buns and chapattis that she sells in various shops around. She said she has been able to run her business effectively because of her involvement in various groups. Through the *upatu*, she has been able to get a significant amount of money to invest in her business. She has hired two girls to help in the business. She also got house furniture from *upatu* contributions. Mama Maiko's household has a distant family farm but the family does not stay there for longer periods of time as other families do. Mama Maiko goes to the distant farm when she has to supervise the labourers. Last season they harvested forty bags of paddy from four acres, part of it was sold and the rest used for own consumption.

Mama Maiko is a member of three groups with different conditions: the Kiwomiki group, the Juataki group and the Jipe moyo utashinda group, with entrance fees of TShs. 10,000, 500 and 1,000, respectively. There are also annual contributions for each group. These groups have women from different tribes and most of the members are aged between 35 and 50. Mama Maiko manages to contribute to all these groups from the money she is making from the business. She said group membership is useful and she is encouraging other women to become members so that they can be assisted in improving their lives.

Case 7.2. Bwana Mlogola: poor, HIV/AIDS-affected, non-group member.

Mr. Mlogola, 36 years old, came to Mkamba in 2001 to find a job. He worked as a seasonal labourer with the Sugar Company but later decided to settle in the village. He is married with one child. The family lives in a rented room with little furniture and without electricity. He has not paid the room rent (TShs. 2,500 month) for the past six months. He got a loan from a friend to buy medicine when he was sick, but has not been able to repay it. He acknowledges that he and his wife are HIV-infected and thinks that their ten months-old son is infected too, because they could not follow the advice they were given during counseling not to breastfeed him. They simply could not afford to buy milk for the baby. Though having cultivated their maize farm last season they had no harvest due to drought. They had to work in their farm themselves because they could not hire labourers or a tractor for ploughing. They depend on odd jobs to make their living, but the man is often unable to work because of frequent bouts of illness. Even the kinds of casual jobs available in the area are too strenuous for him. He thinks that if he could get a driving license, he might be able to get other lighter jobs in the sugar company. Sometimes his wife works on their landlady's plot and gets some food in return. This season she helped with harvesting rice but they are not sure how much they will get.

Bwana Mlogola knows about the groups in the village and appreciates their benefits, but he cannot join because he cannot pay the required contributions. He knows that there is a Wahehe group, the ethnic group he belongs to, but he cannot become a member. The entrance fee (TShs. 3,000) and annual contributions (TShs. 10,000) are too expensive for him. He would also not be able to attend to the group meetings due to lack of time or illness. He attends one of the Protestant churches in the village for spiritual and emotional support. The couple does not receive any practical and material support from their Church. He told me he would not mind telling people about their health status but his wife is worried of the treatment she is going to get once people they know they are infected. She is scared of being laughed at, stigmatized and isolated by other community members. He says: 'Once people know that you are affected they will not even give you a loan because they know you are soon going to die', telling me I am the next person after the counselor to know about their HIV/AIDS status. He does not mind a stranger knowing it. He thinks strangers could offer the possibility for medical and other assistance but not the people in the village. He does not know about SHDEPHA$^+$ in Ruaha. He later visited the organization and was told to go to Ifakara Hospital for CD4 count test for which he had to pay about TShs. 25,000. He did not go because he could not afford the expenses involved, including the fare.

in groups, which offer opportunities for advancement. The case of Hawa (Case 5.6) shows that even an individual in an HIV/AIDS-affected household can become a member of a group and benefit from it, provided the household is relatively well-off. Although the groups do not address the problems brought about by HIV/AIDS, those from affected households who are members enjoy substantial group advantages that non-members do not get, such as lump-sum cash from *upatu* schemes and group help during funerals. However, the increasing incidence of death and illness associated with AIDS puts a strain on group resources (cash, time and labour). Group members feel that it is beyond the group's capability those affected the attention they need. As one of the woman group members says:

> *'Bearing in mind our economic hardship, we cannot deceive ourselves that we are able to give full support to those affected, their demands are so great and our group cannot mobilize enough resources to attend to all.'*

Because men and women may face different barriers to group membership, gender is likely to be another important determinant of group participation. Although Table 7.1 indicates that sex of the respondent does not have significant influence on group membership, there appear to be differences in the types of groups to which men and women belong. From the group inventory it was found that out of 20 groups found in the village 14 comprise women only, 5 are mixed, and only one is exclusively male. Predominantly, women groups are self-help groups that have grown out of local circumstances to meet the specific needs of women, such as burial groups and ROSCAs. Women groups are organized to address day-to-day economic needs and constraints and to improve the household well-being. Most women participate in *upatu* arrangements in which membership conditions are relatively easy to fulfill. More than women, men dominate groups that have substantial resources, but to become a member of those groups involves significant financial contributions. Examples of groups in Mkamba in which men dominate are the sugarcane out-grower production groups and the formally registered saving-and-credit group. These differences show how groups are gendered in nature and that for men and women membership depends on the type of groups. These findings are similar to what Qodquin & Quisumbing (2005) reported in their study of Philippine rural communities.

Despite potential benefits of group involvement, groups may place personal obligations on members that are difficult to meet, especially for the poor and HIV/AIDS-affected households. Some of the non-group members interviewed said they were once members in groups, but the conditions were difficult to fulfill, especially when they had no sufficient income and time for both their households and groups contributions as a woman villager recounts:

> *'It is difficult to get time to go for meetings and have money to contribute to the group, when you have to attend most of the things in your household; you have to strive for your household first.'*

More than half of respondents are not members of a group. Fifty-seven percent of non-members feel that the conditions for membership are difficult to fulfill. About 27 percent said they are fewer groups of their interests, 17 percent mentioned lack of time to participate in group activities and the remaining proportion mentioned lack of information on groups' membership conditions, non-approval by the husband, and sickness as reasons for non-membership.

7.3 Community solidarity

According to Narayan & Pritchett (1999), community social capital is important in determining households' income and ability to cope with social and economic calamities. Nevertheless, communities vary in social capital they have and how they use it to respond to the difficulties poor or HIV/AIDS-affected households face. Community characteristics such as ethnic diversity, presence of groups, NGOs, community programs, volunteering spirit and general trust determine a community's ability to cope. Where social relations are under stress, local organizations often suffer. Many key informants and participants in the focus group discussions remarked that interpersonal relations and community actions are declining due to various socio-economic factors such as economic stress and poverty that make people self-centred and individualistic as they try to survive.

7.3.1 Helping with day-to-day problems

In Mkamba death is an event that triggers collective community participation. In case of a death of a village member, villagers contribute in-kind and cash to facilitate the funeral. Each villager is supposed to contribute at least TShs. 50. Those who contribute are recorded in a special book. There is a separate book for women and men. The books are kept for future reference, from which the information on amount collected and those contributed can be retrieved. For those unable to attend the burial, the designated persons from each hamlet collects contributions from them. Elderly and orphaned households are exempted. The money is used to buy the burial garment (*sanda*) for the corpse, the coffin, and for feeding the mourners before the burial. Before burial, the amount of money collected is announced to the public. However, during informal talks a lot of people complained that in many cases the contributions are collected even after the burial, when cash is no longer needed. They said collecting contributions after the burial creates a loophole for squandering the money. Some of the village leaders said the cash collected after the burial is needed to enable the family to pay the debts in case they borrowed money to cover some of the funeral expenses. There are still cash and in-kind contributions of groups if it concerns the household of a member as well as from *watani* (jokers). Activities at funerals are organized along gender lines. During funerals women who attend bring a bowl (about ¼ kilogram) of maize flour and pieces of fuel wood. While there, women have to fetch water and participate in cooking for the family and the mourners. Men are involved in digging the grave, carrying the coffin to the graveyard and filling the grave with earth. A small group of men is involved in coordinating all the activities for the funeral ceremony.

Those who did not participate in other people's funerals are likely to face sanctions when they have to bury someone themselves. In case of death in their household, very few people will make cash contributions, which may hamper the purchase of important items for burial and the performance of different activities during the funeral. However, an elderly informant said, on humane grounds the villagers may still assist at the burial and later they will have to explain to the family how important good relations with other households are. Regarding people's participation in funerals one village woman lamented that:

> *'So many deaths occur in the village such that you cannot divide yourself to attend to all the funerals. You might be seen as uncooperative but there are just too many.'*

Despite increased deaths in the village people still make efforts to participate in funerals of others knowing they will receive similar treatment when it is their turn. In most cases households cannot meet funeral expenses on their own and participate in other funerals to mobilize social support.

There is no such evidence of community involvement in assisting households facing calamities like illness or food shortage. These problems are considered to be private and a family responsibility. According to the village leaders, although the villagers at first planned to help vulnerable households like those of elderly, widows, orphans and the very poor, they could not do so because it was difficult to mobilize funds from the villagers who were facing similar or other problems. In a few instances, donations from the community were mobilized, but the amount collected did not meet the needs of the vulnerable households and individuals. According to one village leader, it was impossible to decide who has a genuine problem and who has not, because many people report having problems. It is not possible to raise the money for all of them. Although money is still occasionally collected the results are not very good. Some people feel the money is being misused by those assigned to collect it because they do not report to the public how much has been collected and used. This indicates that there is lack of trust among the people.

7.3.2 Community voluntary and compulsory contributions

Communal activities are an important aspect of community life. The ability to work voluntarily together with others for the common good is likely to generate social capital. Volunteering in various collective activities expresses the concern for others and public interests. Volunteering in public-interest activities has been used as an indicator of social capital in this study. Volunteering builds social ties and facilitates collective actions for the common good and is viewed to be at the heart of social capital (Onyx & Leonard, 2002). Participation in voluntary activities may build community social capital by fostering trust among community members and develop social networks and cooperation among community members, which in turn contributes to a cohesive and prosperous community (Putnam, 1993). In the study area participation in collective activities for the public interest is labeled as voluntary work (*Kazi ya kujitolea*). They are considered voluntary because they do not involve financial rewards to those involved. They include a range of activities mainly for the public interest, such as classroom and health centre construction, road maintenance, water-system management and contributing labour to emergency work in case of outbreaks of disease such as cholera. Others include religious and political activities.

For public activities, the contribution of each household in terms of cash and labour is decided at village meetings. Most of these activities are organized by hamlet leaders channeled through ten-cell leaders. A number of household are organized to work together in turns. The ten-cell leaders are responsible for mobilizing people in their jurisdiction to participate in those activities. Participation is compulsory and an attendance register is kept. Those who do not attend without notice are followed up. There are village bylaws on voluntary work. Those who did not attend without good reason are fined according to these bylaws and can be taken to the village court if they fail to pay. Fines are either in cash or in kind. Elderly households are exempted from participating.

Respondents were asked to report on their voluntary work in the past and whether those activities were compulsory or voluntarily. About 91 percent reported participation in communal work, 87 percent of which was compulsory and the remainder voluntary. Religious and political activities are done on a voluntary basis. Classroom and health centre construction and rehabilitation of water points are considered important activities in which the majority of the respondents participated as required. For construction work, each household has to participate by donating money (TShs. 1,500) and making in-kind contributions of locally available building materials such as stones, sand and bricks. Additionally, households have to provide labour to assist the technicians during construction work. The rest of the expenses are covered by the government through a debt relief fund. Respondents' participation in school and health centre construction was very high because of close follow-up by the village authorities. Likewise, the district and central government authorities closely monitor the execution of these activities and the use of funds. Community participation as a development strategy has been emphasized in all national policies. The village has agreed to have obligatory contributions as a way of meeting the requirement for community contribution in order to qualify for grants from various sources. Most of the so-called voluntary work in this context is mandatory though the community refers to them as voluntary. There are differences among communities as to what constitute voluntary activities. Some of the informants were concerned that there had been too much of collective voluntary work and that it is mainly the poor who participate because well-off households may use their influence to avoid participation. Others had a different opinion, saying that it is the community members' responsibility to make sure they have necessary basic services and not rely entirely on the government provisions.

Success or unsuccessful experience with community projects was also used as an indicator of community solidarity in response to various public concerns and problems. The construction and installation of a water system in the village was known as a very successful project. Its success can be explained by the fact that water is a very important need to every one and solving the problem of water shortage requires cooperation. Some projects have not been successful, such as the construction of a village office and a local police post. The projects failed because of poor leadership (40%), political conflicts (27%), and financial problems (13%). Further probing during Focus Group Discussion 6 (see Table 3.2) revealed that these failures were caused by the lack of unity among the community members.

7.3.3 HIV/AIDS community-based interventions

Increasingly communities are recognized to be among the actors in HIV/AIDS prevention, care and mitigation of its impacts. An important aspect of the Tanzanian government's strategy to mitigate the impacts of HIV/AIDS has been to promote and support community-based programs, in both rural and urban areas. It is assumed that communities will develop a variety of ways to cope with the growing AIDS crisis, because communal initiatives are based on the assumption that strength of families and communities is that people will support each other and care for those afflicted and their families. Community members are supposed to be in a position to know who needs help. Those involved are community-based health workers, religious groups, CBOs and NGOs.

The village health workers' post is the lowest level of the health care delivery in the country. It provides preventive services in homes, offers first aid services and acts as a distribution point for items like condoms and oral dehydration salts. Village health care workers are chosen by the village government from among the villagers and are given training. In Mkamba there is one village health care worker in every hamlet. These persons work in collaboration with the village dispensary. They visit those who are known to have chronic illnesses and offer counseling and basic drugs, if available. However, these persons have been operating under difficult conditions and have no first aid kits. They are also demoralized because they are not paid regularly. The village is responsible for their payments and in most cases the village government has to mobilize contributions from the community members, which arc not casy to gct.

As religious organizations are rooted in local communities, they are in an excellent position to mobilize community activities against HIV/AIDS. In other areas religious organizations have been the first to respond to the basic needs of people affected by the disease and indeed have pioneered much of the community-based work. But in Mkamba few people reported getting support from religious groups, which is usually consisting of moral and spiritual support.

HIV/AIDS prevention of mother-to-child transmission is another HIV/AIDS-specific activity facilitated by an international NGO called AXIOS. This project targets all women attending the antenatal clinic. In collaboration with the village dispensary, the program conducts pre-and post-counseling to mothers who attend the antenatal clinic. Those who are willing to be tested do so and are informed about the results. Women, who are found to be HIV-positive, are given a special drug (Nevirapin) when they start experiencing labour pains and Nevirapin syrup to the new-born 72 hours after birth. The mothers are also advised on feeding practices: they should either breastfeed exclusively for six month or not at all. Spouses of those affected are also advised to go for a test but there is very little turn-up. According to nurse in charge of the local dispensary HIV affected-women are not able to tell their partners about their status and to persuade them to go for a HIV test. In most cases the men would accuse their partners for the infection though they might be responsible themselves. Because of women fear such accusations they don't inform their partner. For the mothers it is also difficult to follow the advised feeding practices, as it involves substantial cash resources which most of them do not have.

Widespread awareness on prevention, transmission, management and mitigation of HIV/AIDS is important for the community because it might prevent problems. Peer educators play a major role in raising community awareness. In Mkamba there are twenty peer educators, youths who were mobilized by the village to join the special UNICEF program for Out-of-School Youth. Their main task is to sensitize the community on HIV/AIDS and other STIs. They usually perform different activities, e.g. drama, role-play and singing to make people aware of the dangers and impacts of infection, discuss stigma and discourage traditions and practices that may lead to spread of the disease. Some of the educators have attended seminars on communication and awareness creation.

In contrast to the neighbouring village of Kidatu (see below) apart from awareness programs in Mkamba there are no community initiatives to assist vulnerable households, especially those affected by HIV/AIDS. Some groups assist their members but regular assistance is not guaranteed. Solving domestic problems such as care for the sick and food provision is generally perceived to be the household's responsibility (especially of women or close relatives). One of the village hamlet leaders said:

> *'Even if we give assistance to affected or vulnerable households, which is not easy these days anyway, it is still the household's responsibility to care for its members; no one will leave her/his family to care for others.'*

7.3.4 Comparison with another village

Despite difficulties brought about by various socio-economic changes in Tanzanian society, some communities appear to be somehow better positioned to help people cope than others. To find explanations for these differences, in this section Mkamba village is compared to the neighbouring village of Kidatu.

Kidatu village profile

This village was registered in 1976 as a so-called *Ujamaa* village. The village has a total population of 10,274 people living in three hamlets. According to the village leader, the village population has increased in recent years. Due to population pressure in Mkamba village some of those who came to look for employment and business opportunities have now settled in Kidatu. The village has two primary schools and shares a dispensary with Mkamba village. Most of the villagers have farming plots near the village, although some have distant farming plots. There are also sugarcane out-growers in the village. Although there is a noticeable ethnic diversity, the main ethnic group in the village is Wasagala who are more or less the same as Wapogoro and Wandamba, who are also represented in the village. These ethnic groups share the same culture and perceive themselves as related. Other tribes in Kidatu village are the Wangoni, Wangindo and Wandwewe who are *watani* (jokers) to the Wasagala, who are supposed to live with them as relatives. Historically, these ethnic groups know each other, and in case of problems they used to to help each other. As it is with other parts of Kilombero District, people in Kidatu village have a very strong belief in witchcraft and many people have been taken for cleansing rituals. Kidatu village has a village development fund called MFUMAKI (MFuko wa MAendeleo KIdatu). Funds are generated from the village sugarcane plot of about 60 acres. Since it is difficult to communally work on the farm, the plots are let for hire to individuals and various groups in the area. These groups pay land rent, thus producing a significant income to finance village activities. Another source of revenue is from a mining quarry located in the village.

Discussion with the village leaders and a few informants revealed that there is some collective effort to assist vulnerable and HIV/AIDS-affected households in various ways. Households identified as HIV/AIDS-affected and the very poor are given special treatment when it comes to education and health care services. Orphans of school-age are given uniforms and other school items by the village government. They are not charged for the medical services when visiting public dispensaries. Most of them are known to many villagers. Some of the orphans are fostered by different households which sometimes get financial assistance from the village.

Despite the fact that both villages have similarities in terms of ecological and geographical profile, strong witchcraft beliefs and economic hardship as a result of socio-economic changes, questions arise as to why assistance to HIV/AIDS-affected households is better organized in Kidatu than Mkamba. It was found that Kidatu villagers have very strong bonds and consider themselves as relatives. Interpersonal ties are relatively strong because of perceived strong kinship relations, although also here due to economic change people are less likely to help each other these days. Different from Mkamba, most of the Kidatu inhabitants have been living in the village for a very long time, whereas most of the people in Mkamba village are newcomers. Kidatu village is less diverse in terms of ethnic groups with most people belonging to more or less the same ethnic groups. The communally-owned resources generate income for the village development fund, which makes financial assistance to the needy possible. Good leadership was said to be another factor contributing to common community concerns and working towards solving members' problems. Leaders are committed to make sure that the money collected is used for the purposes of village development and assistance to vulnerable households. The differences found between the two villages indicate that community-level characteristics are important in determining the ability of the villagers to come up with a common plan and actions to help the poor and most vulnerable.

7.4 Trust in the community: myths on community solidarity

Trust is an important component of community-level social capital. Where there is high level of trust, it is likely that associational and collective activities will be supported in the community. During focus group discussions (FGD 6 and 7, see Table 3.2) and informal interviews people expressed their views on declining trust in Mkamba village. In the household survey people were asked to gauge their level of trust in the community by indicating how much they trust their relatives, people from same ethnic group, neigbours and friends as well as the local village government. Fifty-five percent said the level of trust had declined compared to five years ago, and 52 percent attributed this decline to greater economic difficulties. Since many people do not have reliable incomes they are not trusted in matters of money borrowing as stated by ninety-three percent of the respondents. Other reasons mentioned for the decline of trust in the village include selfishness (22%), and witchcraft accusations, ethnic diversity due to population increase, as well as to changes in values, corruption and increased theft (together 26%). All these aspects have undermined trust in the community and lack of solidarity among villagers, which discourages communal activities.

As said above, the issue of witchcraft looms large in the study area. An elderly woman key informant said that in the past witchcraft accusations were between relatives and were solved within the family, but nowadays anybody can be accused of being a witch and that has far-reaching implications. People are reluctant to help others for fear of being accused to be witches. Key informants put forward the following reasons for the increase of witchcraft accusations in the area. First, the village population has grown tremendously, bringing in people from different ethnic backgrounds that are likely not to trust each other. Secondly, some accusations are motivated by jealousy and hatred towards better-off households due to rampant poverty among the people in the area. Third, there are many incidences of prolonged illness and deaths for which witchcraft is used as an explanation. TB and other prolonged illness have always been seen as a witchcraft-induced disease. Ashforth (2001) notes that different from other epidemics, an epidemic such as HIV/AIDS that hits particular persons within a group can easily lead to the suspicion that malicious individuals are pursuing secret evil work. In Mkamba, witchcraft accusations affect trust among the villagers and their proliferation seems to point to collapsing social structures.

7.5 Conclusion: safety nets with holes?

Participation in voluntary groups is commonly used as an indicator for social capital and has been promoted as one of the ways by which the poor can escape from poverty (World Bank, 2000b). Results from this chapter suggest that while it would appear that formal groups can be successful rural institutions, their role should not be overrated because of their exclusive nature and limited capabilities. The very poor and known HIV/AIDS-affected households tend to be barred from membership because of their inability to pay the contributions or because of stigma, or both. Although many discussions of social capital have focused on its positive role for individuals and community, social capital has a dark side (Portes, 1998). The effects of group membership are not always positive. In the study area gender, ethnicity and socio-economic status were evidently criteria for exclusion. Community groups that help to establish beneficial relationships for some individuals may lead to the exclusion of others, who do not have the resources to participate. This means that those most in need are left out and that the claim that all members of the community could benefit from social capital is questionable. As AIDS impacts deepen, households become unable to cope, implying that community assistance is needed. However, the problems of vulnerable households such as food shortage and lack of health care that could have activated community assistance are regarded as family responsibilities. The exclusion of the poor from communal support has been reported in other contexts as well. Sauerborn *et al.* (1996) in their study in Burkina Faso found that as illness occurs in households, the costs are borne by the households on their own and that they rarely get support from the community. Their findings and the findings presented here refute the argument that social capital is a resource for the poor.

The need to fill gaps that are not catered for by government or mainstream development organizations prompted the proliferation of groups in the area. Most of these groups are unregistered and evolved among people with common problems. Despite the increased number of groups in the area, most of them cannot offer sufficient support to their members. They operate in relative isolation and lack structured vertical links to similar or different groups. Bonding social capital was found to be beneficial but not enough to meet most of the household's needs. Lack of bridging social capital results in fewer opportunities for the poor to escape from poverty, as is the case in the study area. I agree with Woolcock & Narayan (2000) that it is a combination of bonding and bridging social capital that allows the communities to confront poverty and take advantage of new opportunities. It was found that there are more women groups than men groups. Most of the activities of the women group aim at accessing resources for household well-being. This proves what has been said that women's social capital profile is more suited to 'getting by' rather than 'getting on' (Lowndes, 2003). There also proved to be differences in the type of groups to which men and women belong. Men are more likely to join production and formal saving and credit groups, because they have the resources needed to become members. It was apparent that women groups in the area work for the improvement of their members' living conditions but do not question dominant gender ideologies and women's subordination. Rankin (2002) urged that the mere formation of women solidarity groups does not guarantee progressive outcomes and may in fact strengthen existing social hierarchies if those groups do not address 'strategic gender needs' (cf. Moser, 1998).

A community's ability to cope with adversity is strongly determined by its ability to act collectively (Adger, 2003). In the literature the positive role of collective actions that is built through repeated interaction in associations is emphasized. According to Moser (1996) and Narayan (1997) communities endowed with rich social networks and civil organizations are more likely to cope successfully with adverse situations than communities without those endowments. In the face of HIV/AIDS, assistance from the community to affected individuals and households has been documented (Mutangadura *et al.*, 1999; Nguthi, 2007). Research findings from Kagera, a region widely studied to investigate HIV/AIDS impacts in Tanzania, show that AIDS has facilitated community-based support networks that enhance community cohesion, but a note of caution is expressed about the possibility of weakened cohesion if the epidemic continues to strike (Tibaijuka, 1997; Rugalema, 1999; Lwihula, 1998). Based on research in Malawi, Mtika (2001) also suggests that when the spread of AIDS reaches a certain threshold level, social capital endowments become unfavorable and reciprocity is undermined, thereby weakening community resistance against AIDS. Findings from this study show that quite a few community-level initiatives emerged in the village in response to the devastating effects of the epidemic. However, assistance offered by groups during illness is limited and a member cannot claim support more than once. Support by groups does not go beyond financial and emotional support and some provision of labour during funerals and festivals.

The study area is experiencing multiple stresses with HIV/AIDS impacts adding to the stress. Community support is no longer effective to meet the multitude of needs resulting from HIV/AIDS epidemic and other socio-economic problems in the area. Economic stress and hardship seem to affect the community in two nearly opposite ways. As individuals and households struggle to make ends meet, they have little time for group and communal activities and concerns. People's preoccupation with of everyday life is dominated by 'getting by'. HIV/AIDS also has a profoundly negative effect on the community's capacity to mobilize people for community actions, since through death and illness HIV/AIDS reduces the number of people who may be involved in community activities. Moreover, because of the clustered nature of the HIV/AIDS impacts it is likely that many individuals and households in the community are directly or indirectly affected, as was aptly expressed by one government official key informant: 'Everyone is affected'. Similarly, Baylies (2002) in her study in Zambia found that AIDS undermines communities and compromises their ability to recover from its consequences. Just as households affected with HIV/AIDS may dissolve, so too may HIV/AIDS-affected communities.

At the community level, the coping ability of affected households very much depends on the community's attitude towards helping needy households, the general availability of resources and the level of community spirit and shared vision. In Mkamba, funerals were found to be the only communal event in which solidarity and cooperation among villagers are expressed. There is a general feeling that community solidarity has declined in the past decades because of economic problems, but also due to lack of trust among community members. A comparison between Mkamba and Kidatu shows different levels of community involvement in helping HIV/AIDS-affected households, which can be explained by Kidatu having more communally-owned resources and less ethnic diversity. The fact that in Mkamba there is more ethnic diversity and many people are not rooted in the area may explain why witchcraft becomes so problematic there. In the whole district, including Kidatu, witchcraft beliefs are very strong but in Mkamba witchcraft accusations seem to have become a destructive force. Similar to what Zak & Knack (2001) and Alasina & La Ferrara (2000) found, different forms of heterogeneity such as ethnic diversity are associated with low trust and participation in community activities. The ability to act collectively requires trust among community members (Durlauf & Fafchamps, 2004), but trust was found to be generally lacking in Mkamba. The findings of this study suggest that it is difficult to mobilize community action in a situation characterized by multiple socio-economic problems and lack of trust. They confirm the notion that deprived communities are also likely to be short of social capital. The findings of this chapter also highlights the need to take into account the history of the community concerned and its distinctive features when assessing HIV/AIDS impacts and designing community-based mitigation interventions.

Chapter 8

General conclusions and discussion

This chapter presents the main findings and conclusions of the study. It is divided into two parts. The first part gives a summary of the answers to the research questions formulated in Chapter 1. The second part addresses theoretical and methodological concerns emerging from the study, and looks at policy implications. The research focused on the way in which people in the village of Mkamba in Tanzania that has a high prevalence of HIV/AIDS, interact and cooperate to solve day-to-day problems and issues of shared concern. The study highlights the dynamic interactions between households and the community and the effects of the epidemic and other forces on these connections. The findings show the interface between interpersonal micro-level social capital and community-level social capital, underscoring the fact that impacts of HIV/AIDS that households experience are intimately linked to the complex ways in which people make their living within specific contexts.

8.1 Conclusions

The conclusions and discussion in the subsequent sections are ordered according to the research questions as formulated in Chapter 1.

8.1.1 Dual disaster: HIV/AIDS and livelihood crisis

Question 1: What are the direct effects of HIV/AIDS on household livelihoods?

The study found that HIV/AIDS is an epidemic with wide-ranging implications for infected individuals and affected households and communities. The impacts extend to the household economy and aspects of social organization. In Chapter 5, the analysis of the impacts of HIV/AIDS on households and livelihoods shows them to be devastating. HIV/AIDS affects the key assets on which households draw for their livelihoods and the scope for responses. Illness and death of household members significantly alter household composition, resources and assets base, and livelihood activities. The case studies reveal that the direct loss of human capital and the diversion of resources and income to caring activities have a critical impact on livelihood activities on which households depend on for securing food and income. HIV/AIDS-affected households require more resources to meet the increasing demands but their production capacity is reduced.

The study found that HIV/AIDS causes and intensifies food insecurity. The presence of household member(s) with prolonged illness, household income, sale of labour were found to influence household food security in a statistically significant way. HIV/AIDS-affected households do not have available labour and cash resources to invest in their farms and other income-generating activities. As a result, they face increased difficulties in ensuring their food security. The evidence from this study shows that food security and HIV/AIDS impacts are bi-directional. On the one hand, as was revealed in the case studies of HIV/AIDS-affected households, AIDS-induced illness and death removes labour and other resources that could have been used in food production and income generation, leading to food insecurity. On the other hand, lack of food leads to malnutrition, which makes infected people more susceptibility to opportunistic infections and leads to earlier onset of full-blown AIDS. This has been documented in the literature (Stillwaggon, 2006) and is illustrated by a case (Case 6.3) in the study. Additionally, food insecurity may drive people to adopt risky survival strategies. Examples reported in the focus group discussions include selling assets (bicycles, household furniture) to buy food and engaging in transactional sex for food and money by women and girls.

It was found that when a household experiences prolonged illness of one or more of its adult household members, it changes its livelihood activities to adapt to the changing labour demands and declining resources. Most of the HIV/AIDS-affected households withdrew from distant farming and resorted to home-based, small-scale activities such as petty trade and gardening, which generally do not yield enough to sustain their livelihoods because of constraints of lack of initial capital and low local purchasing power.

The qualitative findings suggest that the ability of HIV/AIDS-affected households to cope with shock is severely compromised by the depletion of their resources. Poor households with few resources find it hard to respond to the epidemic's effects, to the extent that some households live in destitution. Well-off households affected by HIV/AIDS (Case 5.6) have resources that enable them to cope with the impacts. Therefore, the ability of households to manage the illness and death of one or more adult members depends, among other things, on socio-economic status prior to the presence of HIV/AIDS, availability of household labour (household size and composition), and the ability to minimize loss of assets.

Because of limited access to and control over resources women were found to be especially vulnerable to HIV/AIDS impacts. The qualitative findings show that women bear the brunt associated with HIV/AIDS impacts and other economic crises and shocks, also because the burden of care tends to fall on women. Caring for the sick and orphans has been added to their existing workload, thus reducing their time for productive activities. Increased care demands worsen women's already low access to resources and increase their economic vulnerability. They may engage in risky behaviour to secure income for household needs.

Care provision is continuously challenged in times of HIV/AIDS, because of the increased labour demands due to prolonged illness and orphan care and exhaustion of resources that are necessary to provide care. Provision of adequate care is also hampered by the stigma still attached to the disease. Stigma is manifested by the fact that people distance themselves from and socially exclude persons known or suspected to be infected. Infected women are abandoned by their partners and have to struggle looking after themselves and their family. People with HIV/AIDS are gossiped about and their illness is seen as a result of personal irresponsibility. Because of HIV/AIDS-related stigma, affected households do not get the support they need from their family and from the community.

Young adults' morbidity due to AIDS changes the pattern of intergenerational obligations and responsibilities. As some of the case studies show, instead of being provided for, elderly parents struggle to provide care and support to their sick dying children and orphaned grandchildren. Loss of income, care-related expenses, the reduced ability of caregivers to work, and mounting medical fees push affected households deeper into poverty. Children are forced to acquire adult responsibilities in the event of their parents' illness or death. They become important actors in both care and production, and circumstances force them to work for their food and other necessities. Their involvement in these activities prevents them from going to school.

8.1.2 Degeneration or regeneration of social capital in the face of HIV/AIDS?

Question 2: What is the influence of HIV/AIDS on social capital?

Although illness is at one point a private and individual matter, it has implications for social relationships and functioning. Recourse to social networks is among the known strategies adopted by households and individuals under stress. Households draw on social networks within and outside the extended family and both on individuals and organizations (such as self-help groups) for assistance in times of need. These social relations are very important in building trust, needed to facilitate cooperation among community members. The findings presented in Chapter 6 and 7 demonstrate that in conjunction with other socio-economic changes, HIV/AIDS triggers the breakdown of inter-household reciprocal relations that are vital for individuals and households in times of crises.

Findings from the Kagera region in Tanzania (Lwihula, 1998; Rugalema, 1999; World Bank, 1997; Tibaijuka, 1997), rural Burkina Faso (Sauerborn *et al.*, 1996) and Uganda (Barnett *et al.*, 1995), show that the most important source of assistance to HIV/AIDS-affected households are relatives and local groups. To cope with the financial demands of caring for AIDS patients, new savings-and-credit and mutual aid societies are created. Amuyunzu-Nyamongo and Ezeh (2005) found in Kenya that norms of reciprocity to some extent survived, even in difficult circumstances. Support was extended to others with serious problems such as lack of food. However, in Mkamba community-based support to HIV/AIDS-affected households proved to be very patchy. While reportedly in the past people in the area exchanged labour, food and services, these practices no longer exist. The case studies and focus group discussions revealed that households in need do not get enough labour, food and financial support from the extended family and from other community members. Community assistance is limited to contributions of food and labour to funerals and provision of emotional support. Labour and financial constraints and the stigma associated with HIV/AIDS limit the participation of individuals and households affected by HIV/AIDS in informal social networks and community groups, hence depriving those affected from support.

The family is assumed to be the best venue for providing care and support to HIV/AIDS-infected persons and others affected by the epidemic, but this study has found increasing economic and social pressures reduce its ability to do so. HIV/AIDS impacts have also affected the ability and willingness of extended family members to care for the sick and their survivors, especially children orphaned by HIV/AIDS. The sick and the orphans do not get enough support because their relatives are already too burdened to adequately care for them. Ideally, proximity to relatives enables persons in problems to get emotional and material support. However, it was found that the increasing economic difficulties and migration have led to the dispersal of kinship networks and the deterioration of family support systems, a situation that is aggravated by HIV/AIDS. As community members die and household resources are used for care and funeral expenses, little is left to support those in need, let alone for investing in reciprocal relationships. HIV/AIDS destabilizes reciprocity balances as it kills people at an age where they are expected to engage in reciprocal relationships. For HIV/AIDS-affected villagers who could not get support from their kin, friends and neighbours are the last resort. Though friends and neighbours do provide support to those in need, their assistance proved to be unreliable and irregular.

Lack of interpersonal trust has curtailed social networks and reciprocity relations in Mkamba. Association of AIDS-related illnesses with witchcraft hampers the development of interpersonal trust among community members. The qualitative data shows that support to those with problems is hindered by fear of witchcraft accusation. This has a damaging effect on interpersonal trust, which in turn limits the support one can get from the community members. Furthermore, widespread poverty and ethnic diversity also proved to have a negative effect on interpersonal trust. Poor people have difficulties in borrowing money because they are considered unable to repay their loans. High ethnic diversity in the study area, resulting from its history of association with the sugar cane plantation that has attracted outside labour, was also found to impede trust among community members.

In Mkamba, no community groups evolved to deal with HIV/AIDS impacts. Although the number of groups in the area has increased, no new groups were formed to specifically deal with HIV/AIDS. The groups were established for other purposes and have not incorporated AIDS into their objectives and activities, though the few HIV/AIDS-affected individuals who are a member can still benefit from them. The amount of assistance that community groups provide is generally limited and short-term in nature. For example, in the case of illness members are entitled to assistance only once. In the event of death, support is usually limited to the funeral and burial activities. No assistance could be recorded to vulnerable and HIV/AIDS-affected households that faced problems such as prolonged illness, lack of labour and food insecurity. Such problems, which could have attracted community support, are said to be private and family responsibilities. Key informants also stated that the community does not have the capacity to attend to numerous needs of its members because of poverty.

Though formal and informal networks are generally based on reciprocity and solidarity, there are also inequalities that in most cases are detrimental to the less powerful, such as women and poor households. Age, duration of stay in the village and household income proved to significantly determine membership in groups. Because of lack of resources HIV/AIDS-households and poor households are unlikely to participate in social networks and groups, which in turn affect their access to resources and ability to respond to HIV/AIDS-related and other problems. Compared to men, women were found to participate more in informal social networks. Though women groups help members to 'get by', they were found to command fewer economic resources than men. Moreover, married women's participation in these networks is sometimes restricted by their husbands.

Vulnerability such as caused by HIV/AIDS might foster collective responses among community members, which in turn encourage personal empowerment and social change (Haddad & Gillespie, 2001). The literature has documented cases where the HIV/AIDS epidemic has shown to trigger community responses to help those directly affected (Baylies, 2002; Mtika, 2001; Nnko *et al.*, 2000). Hence, it was expected in this study that people's awareness of experiencing the same hardships would motivate collective action to solve their problems, but the findings prove otherwise. In contrast to a neighbouring village, in Mkamba there are no community-level initiatives for care and support to those directly affected by HIV/AIDS. Lack of communally-owned resources, ethnic diversity and lack of trust in the village are explanatory factors. Even though people may be willing to get engaged in joint action, they do not have the resources to come up with effective community responses. While the strengths and capacities of local communities are often cited as a substantive means to cope with the multiple impacts of HIV/AIDS, in fact their capacities may be inadequate. When many people in a community face economic hardship, the community as a whole will be unable to offer assistance to those in need. Indeed, the study area is confronted with a number of socio-economic problems that significantly reduce the social resources on which households can draw as they seek to secure their livelihoods. As Foster (2005) noted, apart from HIV/AIDS other factors may lead to the collapse of community safety nets, resulting in destitution. In Mkamba, witchcraft accusations and ethnic heterogeneity have weakened community and inter-household mechanisms of cooperation and trust. Additionally migration has led to the decline of mutual exchanges and transfers. This seriously challenges the general statements and expectations about the role of the family and community in helping HIV/AIDS-affected and other vulnerable households. Niehof (2004a) argues that community-based initiatives that are based on a naïve understanding of community are likely to fail.

8.1.3 Implications of changes in social capital for household livelihood vulnerability

Question 3: What are the implications of changes in social capital for household livelihood vulnerability?

As shown by the case studies mobilization of resources within social networks becomes difficult in case of prolonged illnesses and HIV/AIDS-related stigmatization. HIV/AIDS effects strip households off the resources necessary for mutual exchange. The principle of reciprocity on which the functioning of social networks is based, becomes difficult to apply for most of the HIV/AIDS-affected households and individuals. Inability to reciprocate and prolonged need for assistance are discouraging to helping individuals and households in problems. In a context of dwindling household resources and limited assistance from the government, community support would be important but the social capital embedded in the community is eroded in a situation of scarce resources and distrust, as is the case in Mkamba. As the households that make up the community become poor, the effects are also felt at the community level. The community can only function well, if is not deprived of its material and social resources. In the absence of substantial assistance from relatives and friends and community support, most of the HIV/AIDS-affected households have to cope on their own. Loss of assets and break down of support mechanisms due to HIV/AIDS and other socio-economic problems intensify the vulnerability of rural households and communities to other shocks.

8.1.4 Household responses to the changing social capital and increased livelihood insecurity

Question 4: How do households respond to the changes in social capital and increasing livelihood insecurity?

The findings of this study indicate that, unlike what is reported in some studies (e.g. Mutangadura *et al.,* 1999), very few HIV/AIDS-affected households get labour and financial assistance to care for the sick or help in farming from relatives, friends and neighbours. As discussed above, formal and informal social networks cannot provide sufficient support to buffer the crises experienced by most of the HIV/AIDS-affected and other vulnerable households. Immediate family members, particularly women, are to provide support and care without help from the larger kinship network and the community. Support from siblings is also not forthcoming. The support of friends and neighbours is important in the study area because of the dispersal of the members of the kin group due to migration. However, since many friends and neighbours are experiencing similar problems their support is unreliable and inadequate. Households can hardly cope given the weakening of social networks brought about by HIV/AIDS and other socio-economic stress. Limited support from the community compels HIV/AIDS-affected households and individuals to pursue responses that affect their resilience to future shocks.

To compensate for the declining income as a result of increased medical and other household expenses, HIV/IDS-affected households try to get money by either selling assets or draw from their savings. Livelihood activities diversification to non-farm activities is another way households use to mitigate the impacts of HIV/AIDS on labour and income. However, due to stigma some of the HIV/AIDS-affected individuals find it difficult to engage in those activities. People are sometimes reluctant to buy items and services from individuals who are known or suspected to have AIDS. While affected households are doing their best to respond, their ability to continue to do so diminishes. Most of the case studies depict a situation where coping is already under severe strain. The ability of poor households to deal with the multiple losses arising from HIV/AIDS is pushing members increasingly into desperate and risky situations. When households respond to the epidemic impacts by withdrawing from distant farming, selling assets, marrying off their daughters at an early age, or taking their children from school, future household livelihood and well-being are compromised. Households are trying to manage the impacts of HIV/ AIDS in a situation where other problems exist. HIV/AIDS amplifies these problems and deepens the existing crisis with regard to food and income insecurity.

The profound social and economic effects of the epidemic experienced by the households in this study challenge the usefulness of the concept of coping in the wake of HIV/AIDS. The concept seems hardly applicable in a situation where households are deprived to the extent that they cannot even meet the basic needs of their members. Household responses indicate that they are just struggling, not coping (cf. Rugalema, 2000). Barnett & Whiteside (2002) also note that the concept of coping has severe limitations. Marais (2005, quoted in Gillespie, 2006) notes that since coping is an externally applied value judgment it may or may not correspond to what is actually happening. In Mkamba, many households and the community they are part of actually do *not* cope. While it is generally assumed that HIV/AIDS-affected households cope by relying on their social networks, the findings from this study show that social networks do not provide sufficient and reliable support to help affected households sustain their livelihoods. The affected households in the study area belong to the category of the households with weaker safety nets in the figure presented by Donahue *et al.* (2001: 9) that 'fall through' the vulnerability threshold.

8.2 Theoretical and methodological implications of the research

8.2.1 Social capital

Reciprocal arrangements for sharing of available resources through gifts, loans of cash, food, and labour between relatives and community members have been documented as an important way for people to access resources and cope with problems. Formal and informal social networks are expected to play a significant role in reducing household vulnerability. However, these assumptions have not been systematically challenged in relation to the effects of HIV/AIDS on social capital in Tanzanian communities. The way the concept of social capital has been used in the literature does little to explain the conditions that facilitate or impede the building and maintenance of social capital. This study contributes to the extension of knowledge in this regard. It shows that social capital is a resource that one has to invest in to able to benefit from. Vulnerable households are unable to maintain their participation in social networks for lack of resources to invest in them, which deprives them of support from these networks. The values and norms underpinning these social networks seem to be changing as well. This is indicated by statements of participants in the focus group discussions and key informants about a household's economic problems being a private matter and increasing individualization. HIV/

AIDS combined with other factors have brought about changes in social networks and social norms. HIV/AIDS-related economic hardship, loss of income, migration, changes in familial values and in relations, witchcraft accusations and HIV/AIDS-related stigma, all limit the support vulnerable and HIV/AIDS-affected households can get from their social networks and the community. This may have induced normative change in the sense that one should not expect such support anymore.

The question is to what extent expectations are also changing with regard to kinship support. The research findings show how the foundations on which kinship support is based are being threatened by HIV/AIDS and other factors. Kinship relations are seen as a special category of social relationships which are characterized by feelings of solidarity, obligation and moral claims. When respondents in the survey were asked to name where they got or are likely to get support, most people identified relatives. This shows that in the study area kinship ties remain central in terms of potential for social support. However, empirical evidence from the case studies reveals the weakening of family ties and a diminishing role of kinship relations because of socio-economic change. Moral obligations to support kin are now operating in a context that curtails their realization. For most people support from relatives is not assured and assistance to HIV/AIDS-affected individuals from kin not forthcoming. The geographical distance between members of the extended family due to migration and the inability of many to meet the expectations and obligations attached to kinship ties are determining factors in this. For frequent exchange of care, food and other necessities close proximity is required. In a situation where people have moved in and relatives are not living close by, friendship becomes a vital part of an individual's network. To some people, friends and neighbours are now more important than their biological relatives. As a Swahili proverb says: 'A friend is better than a relative' (*rafiki ni bora kuliko ndugu*).

Apart from the discrepancy between people's expectations about and the reality of support provided by relatives, HIV/AIDS leads to a reversal of the normative model as regards the flow of support between elderly parents and adult children. At a time when they could expect old-age support from their adult children, when an adult son or daughter gets AIDS elderly parents take the care of their sick child and the grandchildren upon them. Even though they may regard the situation as anomalous and may bitterly comment upon it (cf. Case 5.4), they still do it. Finch & Mason (1993) argue that kinship norms of morality are not a 'blue print' of what relatives should and will do for each other and, as could be observed in Mkamba, that economic constraints may hinder support among kin. The question is to what extent a prolonged inability to comply with normative kinship obligations will lead to changes in family values and the normative underpinnings of kinship relations. As Carsten (2004) notes, the value of kinship should be placed in the context of the life course. Though kinship relations represent claims that can be mobilized, reciprocity is involved here as well. Qualitative data shows that extended family members may provide support in times of need if there have been earlier investments in the relationship concerned or if they can expect assistance when they need it.

As with other kinds of capitals, social capital is not equally available to all. It was evident during the study that social networks generate exclusion alongside solidarity, which is why it cannot be seen as panacea to all social and economic problems in communities (cf. Adler & Kwon, 1999; Portes, 1998). Poor households and most of the HIV/AIDS-affected households have limited social networks because of their inability to reciprocate and the stigma attached to their status. The study shows that differences with regard to income and gender intersect with unequal access to social capital. This study also highlights the dynamics between social capital and other assets necessary for livelihoods generation, showing that lack of social capital prevents people from accessing other livelihood resources.

Community social capital

According to Grootaert & Van Basterlaer (2002) social capital should be dealt with at micro, meso and macro-level, but the interface between the three levels has not been widely investigated. This study sheds some light on these linkages. The findings indicate that what is taking place at the micro-level influences the meso-level environment, while the norms and values that underpin social interaction reflect meso-level and macro-level values. Individual or household actions at the micro-level can result into aggregate positive collective action or unintended negative effects (Brons *et al.*, 2007). The collective effects feed back on individual households, which may or may not improve their livelihoods. For example, people in study area were generally found to have weak ties with their kin, friends and neighbours. Poor and HIV/AIDS affected households were generally found to have weakened social networks. This effect of declining micro-level social capital is also felt at the community (meso) level, leading to lack of cooperation and trust among community members. Unlike the people in a neighbouring village and in a village in Kagera (Rugalema, 1999), people in the study area have not been able to devise any community-level mechanism to respond to the HIV/AIDS impacts on affected households.

The community provides an important context within which social support relations evolve, but HIV/AIDS mortality and morbidity impoverish households and deprive communities of individuals who could otherwise engage in community activities. In Mkamba, socio-economic factors such as widespread poverty, ethnic diversity and witchcraft beliefs affect people's relations and the way they try to cope with the various problems. It was found that the influx of people from other areas has resulted in ethnic heterogeneity which seems to have undermined interpersonal trust, making it difficult for the people to work on a common agenda. This finding corroborates the results of a large-scale investigation into migration-induced ethnic diversity and community cohesion by Robert Putnam. Putnam (2007: 149) concludes: '[Ethnic] diversity seems to trigger *not* in-group/out-group division, but anomie or social isolation' (italics in the original). Key informants and participants in the focus group discussions attributed the lack of community solidarity partly to ethnic diversity. Case study 6.3 also shows that even those from the same ethnic group do not offer support to each other. In multi-ethnic communities where people are not rooted in the area like in Mkamba, it is difficult to build networks of trust and strengthen civil society. The proliferation of witchcraft suspicion and accusations also both reflects and leads to deterioration of trust and curtails social interaction. Even though most people are aware that HIV/AIDS is not caused by witchcraft, they still associate misfortunes that are difficult explain such as prolonged illness with it. Distrust at the interpersonal level is extended to the community level, affecting the way people can work together to solve their problems. Collective actions are only possible in a community with sufficient level of trust.

Although the village in Kagera (Rugalema, 1999) and the villages of Kidatu and Mkamba are all embedded in the same macro institutional framework, they vary in the way they mobilize themselves to assist HIV/AIDS-affected and other vulnerable households. Such variation can be explained by the way meso-level social capital operates. Though also in Kagera and Kidatu social networks are strained because of HIV/AIDS impacts and other factors, unlike in Mkamba in these villages people maximize informal contact among relatives, neighbours and friends, which in turn strengthens trust and common values to provide a basis for resilience in problematic times. The quality of social ties among community members and the presence of conditions that promote cooperation and adequacy of resources determine the ability of a community to collectively solve its problems. This shows that any given problem needs to be investigated at both micro- and meso-level in order to arrive to a complete understanding of how social capital works.

8.2.2 Revisiting the household as a unit of analysis

In this study the concept of household has been used to refer to a group of people who occupy the same dwelling that takes care of resource management and the primary needs of its members. Household boundaries are understood to be permeable and household composition changing over time. It was found that in the context of HIV/AIDS, spatial proximity and day-to-day interaction are important in coping with AIDS illnesses and other impacts. Although there may be support from non-household members, it is the household members who are present on daily basis to provide care for the sick by nursing, preparing meals, doing laundry, shopping, and so on. In view of the immediate needs of AIDS patients and their caregivers, households are well described in terms of their functions and the quality of support among their members. Therefore, a household can be defined as a closely-knit web of relations among persons who live together and provide for each other on day-to-day basis. A household is a site of exchange and support relations that is relatively reliable and durable. This definition helps to resolve the issue of household boundaries, as it only includes members who mutually provide for basic needs on daily basis. This does not make the household a closed unit, since household members are part of social networks beyond their own household. Other relations beyond the households can be considered support relations, which this study has found to be less reliable.

For HIV/AIDS research it has been proposed to look beyond the household as a unit of analysis. Müller (2004a;b) suggests a need for a thorough investigation on the wider usefulness and applicability of cluster analysis in studying HIV/AIDS impacts. Although this study did not use the cluster as the unit of analysis, its findings shed some light on this matter. Acknowledging that households are rarely self-contained productive units and that households maintain links with other households, the study moved beyond the household by looking at how households and individuals are integrated in social networks and how they cope with AIDS impacts and other socio-economic challenges within such networks. However, evidence provided by this study and elsewhere (Heuveline, 2004; Desmond *et al.*, 2000) indicates that it is within the HIV/AIDS-affected households that the intense impacts of AIDS epidemic are experienced, in many cases without these households receiving significant support from other households. Even though, through overlapping social relations HIV/AIDS effects may spread to several households, the effects are most pointedly felt by households of HIV-positive people, households that experienced HIV/AIDS-related deaths and those caring for AIDS orphans. Therefore, the household is still the most important context for meeting people's daily needs and providing care for children and the sick (cf. Niehof, 2004c). It is apparent from the case studies (e.g. Case 5.4 and Case 6.1) that affected households do not get any substantial support to care for the sick from beyond their own household and has to struggle by themselves, despite having a number of relatives and friends. Therefore, the use of clusters as the unit of analysis in assessing HIV/AIDS impacts and coping responses does not seem to have an added value in a context like that of the village of Mkamba.

Since HIV/AIDS disrupts established patterns of household life and ways of making a living, in a context of HIV/AIDS households undergo continual change with regard to their composition, entitlements, division of labour and decision-making. As prime-aged adults die, new forms of household emerge such as child- and elderly-headed households, most of which are failing to generate secure livelihoods (Cases

5.1, 5.2, 5.3 and 6.2). This study, albeit based on a relatively small sample, reveals the HIV/AIDS-induced mobility patterns (Cases 5.1, 5.4, 6.1 and 6.2). Return of sick young adults (previously living elsewhere) to their parental household for care entails re-organization of the household resources to cater for their needs. This shows the dynamic nature of household composition. Households are actually fragile and unstable in times of HIV/AIDS. However, as argued above, replacing the household as the unit of analysis by the cluster is not a solution. HIV/AIDS changes household membership and roles with implications on how interventions should be formulated. The dynamics of household structures and composition in the context of HIV/AIDS need to inform the operational definition of household when designing interventions, so that new household forms can be accommodated.

8.2.3 Methodological notes

Incorporating the temporal dimension in studies of HIV/AIDS impacts (Gillespie & Kadiyala, 2005) and household processes (Pennartz & Niehof, 1999) is crucial to capture the dynamics of interactions between HIV/AIDS and livelihoods. The current study could have benefited from panel data to add more value to the research findings. A longitudinal study using both qualitative and quantitative methods could have captured better the local dynamics of HIV/AIDS impacts. It would also have provided more information on micro socio-economic trends, households' ability to cope, and the complex causal relationships involved. However panel data sets are costly and take time to generate. A longitudinal approach to the subject matter of this study would have to include the variables of household composition, assets portfolio, livelihood activities, social support relations, and coping responses.

In this study a discrepancy could be observed between quantitative and qualitative findings with regard to the topics of HIV/AIDS, food security and social support, which could be attributed to two factors. First, in a survey there is a tendency for people to give socially desirable or normatively biased answers, while in in-depth interviews or in less personal focus group discussions they are more likely to report actual behaviour and conditions. This may explain the discrepancy between what respondents reported on issues regarding AIDS, food security and support from relatives and neighbours in the household survey and the information on these topics obtained through observation, case studies, focus group discussions and key informants. Second, operationalization of complex concepts such as social capital and food security is not easy and may not capture all the important dimensions. The complex interactions between the dimensions add to the difficulty of finding valid measures or indicators for such concepts. Qualitative methods complemented survey data by revealing the complex realities of how social capital is generated or eroded in a situation of increasing vulnerability. They enhance the understanding of household processes that are difficult to measure and can provide a picture of actual household responses in dealing with decline in household resources. The story of *'the stone in the cooking pot'* illustrates how revealing information obtained by qualitative methods can be. But to be entrusted with such sensitive and personal information the researcher has to stay in the study area for a longer period of time. The data obtained by quantitative methods could shed light on the relationships between socio-economic aspects and other variables. Thus, the study confirms the need for integrating qualitative and quantitative approaches in HIV/AIDS research. Triangulation is not only as a means for validation, but also helps to gain a deeper understanding of the phenomenon under study.

It was also found that the definition of HIV/AIDS-affected households is a problematic issue. In this study HIV/AIDS-affected households were defined to include households with chronically ill members, had experienced deaths, and/or had taken in orphans. However, the effects of HIV/AIDS vary substantially between and within these groups. Households that have taken in orphans may be relatively well-off and by taking in orphans might add significantly to their household labour potential, which amounts to a positive effect. By using this hybrid definition it was difficult to observe statistically significant effects of the epidemic on variables such as food security, which could be observed when only households with chronically ill members were taken as a separate category. Analysis of effects at different stages of HIV/AIDS impacts is more informative, as the narratives of the case studies show. However, to get statistically significant evidence of the different effects of HIV/AIDS at different stages of impacts would require a large, stratified sample that is difficult to realize because it presupposes information that is rarely available.

8.3 Implications for policies and interventions

The research findings have elucidated the complex interactions between HIV/AIDS, social capital, food security, gender and livelihood and have provided insights on the processes and dynamics involved. But as Barnett (2006) rightfully cautions, easy generalization about HIV/AIDS impacts and processes may lead to inappropriate responses. Because of the fact that HIV/AIDS impacts and social capital are context-specific, the lessons learnt from this study are applicable to areas that are comparable to the study area. When household and community resources are already strained, as in Mkamba, there are no quick fixes to alleviate the economic and social impacts of HIV/AIDS. As Stillwaggon (2006) argues, the interactions between biological, social, economic and environmental factors that comprise the ecology of poverty shape the spread and impacts of HIV/AIDS. This study has shown that the limits to household and community responses stem from the nature of HIV/AIDS and from the particular socio-economic and cultural features of the community concerned.

Moreover, the impacts of the epidemic on those affected differ according to their personal, economic and social circumstances. Therefore, policies and interventions should be holistic and not just address the immediate effects but also take into account important contextual circumstances and underlying causes to HIV/AIDS susceptibility and vulnerability.

Current policies tend to emphasize home-based care for HIV/AIDS-infected people and community-based action, but – as this study shows – the inability of communities like Mkamba to cope with the growing demands for support prevents the full and effective implementation of such initiatives. In such circumstances community-level responses to AIDS cannot be comprehensive enough to address the many effects of the epidemic and other shocks. Because the inability of the community to meet the needs of its vulnerable members is limited, care responsibilities are left to families and, notably, women to shoulder. Little has been done to strengthen the provision of support by communities to vulnerable households. There is a need for joint and coordinated interventions by non-governmental and governmental institutions to help communities cope with the problems created by HIV/AIDS, instead of assuming their ability to do so.

It is necessary to strengthen existing community groups such as women groups, burial groups and saving groups, to enable them to provide the necessary assistance needed by individuals and households to cope with the epidemic and other shocks. Strengthening ties between a diversity of groups in the community should be encouraged to facilitate collective action in response to the crisis. In a multi-ethnic community like Mkamba the role of jokers can be strengthened to help others cope with insecurities. Lack of disclosure of positive HIV-status for fear of stigma tends to mask the magnitude of the epidemic. There is an urgent need to break the silence. Openness will reveal the extent of the problem, thus motivating the broader community to devise appropriate interventions to assist the large numbers of affected households. It is important to foster social relations between affected individuals and households and other community members to secure care and reduce stigmatization in order to enable collective actions.

Clear links have been shown between the pattern of HIV/AIDS impacts and gender inequalities. With the gendered division of labour within households as it is, the impacts of AIDS at household level are profoundly gendered. This suggests that existing development approaches may need to be re-examined in the light of this fact. It is therefore important that HIV/AIDS problems be addressed from a different angle. Gender-sensitive, community-based interventions for coping with the impacts of HIV/AIDS are essential to enable women manage HIV/AIDS impacts. Addressing women's strategic needs is possibly the most effective strategy in reducing susceptibility and vulnerability to HIV/AIDS and enhancing the capabilities of women to cope with the consequences of HIV/AIDS and other shocks. Strategies to reverse women's social and economic disadvantages will enable women to cope more effectively with the impact of AIDS.

Currently, most of the AIDS interventions in Tanzania are short-term and fail to recognize the systemic and long-term nature of the epidemic, which underscores the need for dynamic, diverse, and long-term responses. Interventions are needed both to curb the spread of HIV and mitigate its impacts. Strategies and programs designed to reduce susceptibility to HIV infection should aim at poverty reduction by supporting livelihoods, strengthening food security, enhancing nutrition and health, easing the burden of women, and addressing the issue of orphans. While prevention and curative care are important, there is a need for material support to affected households to mitigate HIV/AIDS impacts and prevent people from becoming destitute. Given that HIV/AIDS impacts are more felt at the household level and force households to draw on their assets to cushion the shock, there is a need to strengthen their economic base and provide them with the means to protect their assets in order to increase resilience to the impacts of AIDS.

This study has shown the weakness of community-based support systems and highlighted the need for safety-nets to support vulnerable groups. Given the limited capacity of poor households to survive livelihood shocks and stresses by drawing on their own meager resources, there is an urgent need for public intervention. The introduction of welfare programs offering benefits to specifically targeted groups is important in the short- and medium-term to mitigate certain aspects effects of the epidemic, for example by ensuring food security and making sure that children of affected households can attend school. I concur with Kakuru (2006) who proposes the provision of free lunches at school to keep children in school, instead of them taking time off or dropping-out altogether to fend for their own personal and school needs. In the long-term, continued efforts at addressing the structural causes of poverty, such as promotion of gender equality, improved educational opportunities and job creation, are important in an era of HIV/AIDS.

Finally, there are pertinent issues that need further study, so that policies, strategies and interventions can be designed to strengthen community support systems and care for vulnerable HIV/AIDS-affected households. Community abilities to mitigate the impacts of HIV/AIDS need to be further explored. Detailed comparative studies including areas with different livelihoods and HIV/AIDS prevalence rates may provide insights about the ways social capital is generated and used in different contexts. Research is also needed to find ways to promote community responses to HIV/AIDS and other shocks. Much remains to be understood about how community organizations can be best supported to develop their social capital and coping capacity.

References

Adams, A. (1993), Food insecurity in Mali: Exploring the role of the moral economy. *IDS Bulletin* 24 (4): 41-51.

Adger, N.W. (2003), Social capital, collective action and adaptation to climate change. *Economic Geography* 79(4): 387-404.

Adler, P.S. & S.W. Kwon (1999), *Social Capital: The Good, the Bad, and the Ugly*. Available at SSRN: http://ssrn.com/abstract=186928 or DOI: 10.2139/ssrn.186928 (Accessed on 21/1/2007: 1345).

Agarwal, B. (1990), Social Security and the Family: Coping with Seasonality and Calamity in Rural India. *Journal of Peasant Studies* 17 (3): 341-412.

Agarwal, B. (1991), Social security and family: Coping with seasonality and calamity in rural India. In: E. Ahmad, J. Dreze, J.Hills & A. Sen (Eds.) *Social security in Developing countries*. Oxford: Clarendon Press, pp. 171-246.

Agarwal, B. (1992), Gender relations and food security: coping with seasonality, drought and famine in South Asia. In: L. Beneria & S. Feldman (Eds.) *Unequal Burden, Economic Crises, Persistent Poverty and Women's Work*. Boulder, San Francisco and Oxford: Westview Press, pp. 181-218.

Agarwal, B. (1997), Bargaining and gender relations within and beyond the household. *Feminist Economics* 3(1): 1-51.

Alasina, A. & E. La Ferrara (2000), Participation in heterogeneous communities. *Quarterly Journal of Economics* 115(3): 847-904.

Ali, A. (2005), *Livelihood and food security in rural Bangladesh. The role of social capital*. PhD Thesis Wageningen University.

Amuyunzu-Nyamongo, M. & A.C. Ezeh (2005), A qualitative assessment of support mechanisms in informal settlements of Nairobi, Kenya. *Journal of Poverty* 9(3): 89-107.

Anderson, M., F. Bechhofer & S. Kendrick (1994), Individual and Household strategies. In: M. Anderson, F. Bechhofer & J. Gershuny (Eds.) *The social and Political economy of the Household*. Oxford: Oxford University Press, pp. 19-67.

Anderson, M.D. & J.T. Cook (1999), Community food security: Practice in need of theory. *Agriculture and Human Values* 16: 141-150.

Ardener, S. (1995), Women making money go round: ROSCAs revisited. In: Ardener, S. & S. Burman (Eds.) *Money-go-round: The importance of rotating saving and credit associations for women*. Oxford, Washington D.C: Berg, pp. 1-19.

Armstrong, A. (1997), Law and the family in Southern Africa. In: A. Adepoju (Ed.) *Family Pupolation and Development in Africa*. Zed books, pp. 183-202.

Appleton, S. (1996) Women-headed household and household welfare: an empirical deconstruction for Uganda. *World Development* 24(12): 1811-1827

Arrow, K. (1999), Observations on social capital. In: P. Dasgupta & I. Serageldin (Eds.) *Social Capital: A Multifaceted Perspective*, Washington DC: The World Bank, pp. 3-5.

References

Ashforth, A. (2001), AIDS, Witchcraft, and the problem of power in post-Apartheid South Africa. *The Occasional Papers number 10* of the School of Social Science, Institute of Advanced Study Princeton University.

AVISO (2004) *An information bulletin on global environmental change and human security.* The Global Environmental Change and Human Security project (GECHS) Issue No. 13.

Baerends, E.A. (1994), *Changing kinship, family and gender relationship in Sub-Saharan Africa.* Leiden Women and Autonomy Centre (VENA), Leiden University.

Bagachwa, M.S.D. (1997), The rural informal sector in Tanzania. In: D. Bryceson & V. Jamal (eds) *Farewell to Farms: De-agrarianisation and employment in Africa.* Aldershot: Ashgate Publishing, pp. 137-154.

Barnett, T. & P. Blaikie (1992), *AIDS in Africa: Its present and future impact.* London: Belhaven Press.

Barnett, T., J. Tumushabe, G. Bantebya, R.S. Sebuliba, J. Ngasongwa, D. Kapinga, M. Ndelike, M. Drinkwater, G. Mitti & M. Haslwimmer (1995), The social and economic impact of HIV/AIDS on farming systems and livelihoods in rural Africa: Some experience and lessons from Uganda, Tanzania and Zambia, *Journal of International Development* 7:1-22.

Barnett, T. & A. Whiteside (1999), HIV/AIDS and development: Case studies and a conceptual Framework, *The European Journal of Development Research* 11 (2): 200-234.

Barnett, T., A. Whiteside & J. Decosas (2000), The Jaipur Paradigm: a conceptual framework for understanding social susceptibility and Vulnerability to HIV, *South African Medical Association Journal* 90(11): 1098-1101.

Barnett, T., A. Whiteside & C. Desmond (2000), The social and economic impact of HIV/AIDS in poor countries: A review of studies and lessons. New York: UNAIDS.

Barnett, T. & G. Rugalema (2001), *Health and nutrition emerging and reemerging issue in developing countries.* Washington DC: IFPRI.

Barnett, T. & A. Whiteside (2002), *AIDS in the Twenty-first Century: Disease and Globalization.* New York: Palgrave Macmillan.

Barnett, T. & A. Whiteside (2002), Poverty and HIV/AIDS: Impact, Coping and Mitigation Policy. In: C. Giovanni Andrea (Ed.) *AIDS, Public Policy and Child Well-Being.* Florence, Italy: UNICEF.

Barnett, T. (2006). HIV/AIDS, Nutrition, and Food Security: Looking to Future Challenges. In: S. Gillespie (Ed.) *AIDS, poverty, and hunger: Challenges and responses,* pp: 341-349. Washington, D.C.: IFPRI.

Baylies, C. (2002), The impacts of AIDS on rural Households in Africa: A shock like any other? *Development and Change* 33(4): 611-632.

Baylies, C. & J. Bujra (2000), *AIDS, sexuality and gender in Africa, collective strategies and struggles in Tanzania and Zambia.* London: Routlegde.

Beauclerk, J. & S. Heap (2003), Civil society-state relationships: Models and actualities. In: B. Pratt (Ed.) *Changing expectations? The concept and practice of civil society in international development.* INTRAC, NGO Management and Policy Series No 16, pp: 11-30.

Bebbington, A. (1999), Capitals and capabilities: A framework for analyzing peasant viability, rural livelihoods and poverty. *World Development* 27(12):2021-2044.

Berger, R.L. (1996), Human behaviour throughout the life course. In: R.L. Berger, J.T. McBran, & M.J. Rifxis (Eds.) *Human behaviour: A perspective for helping professionals.* New York: Longman Publishers.

Berger-Schimitt, R. (2000), Social cohesion as an aspect of the quality of societies: Concept and measurement. *EuReporting working paper No. 14.* Mannheim: Centre for Survey Research and Methodology (ZUMA), Social Indicators Department.

Bernard, H.R. (2002), *Research methods in anthropology: Qualitative and quantitative approaches.* Walnut Creek, Lanham, New York, Oxford: Altamira Press.

Berry, S. (1993), No condition is permanent: The social dynamics of agrarian change in Sub-Saharan Africa. Madison: University of Winsconsin Press.

Beuchelt, T., I. Fischer, H, Korff & G. Buchenrieder (2005), Social Networks as means of information exchange and risk-management. A case study from Northern Vietnam. A paper presented in International Agricultural Research for Development, Stuttgart-Hohenheim October 11-13, 2005. Germany.

Bharat, S., P. Aggleton & P. Tyrer (2001), *India: HIV and AIDS-related discrimination, stigmatization and denial.* Geneva. UNAIDS.

Bitende, S.N., A. Njombe & Z.S. Semgalawe (2001), Women and food security in poverty reduction: A brief overview of Tanzania. TSAP Proceedings 28.

Blaikie, P., T. Cannon, I. Davis & B. Wisner (1994), At Risk: Natural Hazards, People's Vulnerability and Disasters. London: Routledge.

Bonnard, P. (2002), HIV/AIDS mitigation: Using what we already know. Food and Nutrition Technical Assistance, Technical note No. 5. Washington DC: Food and Nutrition Technical Assistance Project, Academy for Educational Development.

Bookawalter, J.T. & J.M. Warner (2001), Power and bargaining in intra-Household resource allocation: Race, class and gender in South Africa. http:// www.umt.edu/ econ/ papers/ Jeffpaper3.pdf (accessed on 21/02/2007: 1010)

Booth, D., F. Lugangira, P. Masanja, A. Mvungi, R. Mwaipopo, J. Mwami & A. Redmayne (1993), *Social, Economic and Cultural Change in Contemporary Tanzania, A People Oriented Focus.* Stockholm: SIDA

Booysen, F.R. & T. Arntz (2003), The methodology of HIV/AIDS impacts studies: a review of current practices. *Social Science and medicine* 56:2391-2405.

Boserup, E. (1970), *Women's Role in Economic Development.* London: Allen and Unwin.

Boserup, E. (1998), Population and the status of women in rural development. In: P. Demeny and G. McNicoll (Eds.) *The Earthscan Reader in Population and Development.* London: Earthscan.

Bossart, R. (2003), In the city, everybody only cares for himself: social relations and illness in Abidjan, Cote d'Ivoire. *Anthropology and medicine* 10(3): 343-359.

Bossert, A. (1988), Formal and informal social security a case study of Tanzania. In: F. Von Benda-Beckmann *et al.,* (Eds.) *Between Kinship and the State. Social Security and Law in Developing Countries.* Dordrecht: Foris Publications, pp. 211-228.

Bourdieu, P. (1985) The forms of capital. In: J. Richardson (Ed.) *Handbook of theory and research for the sociology of education.* New York: Greenwood, pp. 241-258.

Bourque, L.N. (1997), Making space: Social change, identity and the creation of boundaries in the Central Ecuadorian Andes. *Bulletin of Latin American Research* 16(2): 153-167.

Bowie, B., M. Tobias & T. Williams (1996), The private costs of HIV/AIDS. *New Zealand Medical Journal 109:*51- 54.

Bradley, C. & T. Weisner (1997), Introduction: Crisis in the African family. In: T.S. Weisner, C. Bradley, P.L. Kilbride, A.B.C. Ocholla-Ayayo, J. Akong'a & S. Wandibba (Eds.) *African families and the crisis of social change.* Westport CT: Bergin and Garvey, pp. xix - xxxii.

Braun, V.J. (1991), Social security in Sub-saharan Africa: Reflection on policy challenges. In: E. Ahmad, J. Dreze, J. Hills & A. Sen (Eds.) *Social security in Developing countries.* Oxford: Clarendon Press, pp. 395-414.

Brons, J., T. Dietz, A. Niehof & K. Witsenburg (2007), Dimensions of vulnerability of livelihoods in less-favoured area: interplay between the individual and the collective. In: R. Ruben, J. Pender & A. Kuyuenhoven (Eds.) *Sustainable Poverty Reduction in Less-favoured Areas.* Wallingford: CAB International, pp. 91-110.

Brown, C. & A.P. Thakur (1997), *Kinship, Marriage and the Family.* Accra: Ghana University Press.

Bruce R.L., J.J. Bull & F.M. Stewart (2001), Epidemiology, evolution, and future of the HIV/AIDS pandemic. *Emerging Infection Diseases* 7: 505-511.

Bryceson, D.F. (1997), Farewell to farms: De-agrarianisation and employment in Africa. Aldershot: Ashgate Publishing.

Bryceson, D.F. (2002), The scramble in Africa: Reorienting rural livelihoods. *World Development* 30(5): 725-739.

Caldwell, J.C. (1997), The impact of the African AIDS epidemic. *Health Transition Review* 7 (Supplement 2):169-188.

Carsten, J. (2004), Introduction: Cultures of relatedness. In: J. Carsten, (Ed.) *New approaches to the study of kinship.* Cambridge, New York and Melbourne: Cambridge University Press, pp. 1- 36.

Carter, M.R. & J.A. Maluccio (2003), Social capital and coping with economic shocks: An analysis of stunting of South African children. *World Development* 31(7): 1147-1163.

Chambers, R. (1989), Vulnerability, coping and policy, *IDS Bulletin* (Vulnerability: How the Poor Cope) 20(2): 1-7.

Chambers, R. & G. Conway (1992), Sustainable rural livelihoods: practical concepts for the 21st century. *IDS Discussion Paper no. 296.* Brighton, UK: Institute of Development Studies.

Chant, S. (2003), Female household headship and the feminization of poverty: Facts, fictions and forward Strategies. *New working paper series,* Gender Institute, London School of Economics and Political science.

Chayanov, A.V. (1986), *The Theory of Peasant Economy.* Manchester: Manchester University Press.

Cheal, D. (1989) Strategies of resource management in household economies: Moral economy or political economy. In: R. Wilk (Ed.) *The household economy: reconsidering the domestic mode of production.* Boulder, San Francisco, London: Westview Press, pp. 11-22.

Christiaensen, L. & R.N. Boisvert (2000), Measuring household food vulnerability: case evidence from Northern Mali. *Working Paper 2000-05*. Cornell University: Department of agriculture, Resource, and Managerial Economics.

Christiaensen, L. & K. Subbarao (2005), Toward an understanding of household vulnerability in rural Kenya. *Journal of African Economies* 14-4: pp: 520-558.

Clay, C.D. & H.K. Schwartzweller (1991), Introduction: Researching household strategies. *Research in rural sociology and Development* 5: 1-11.

Cleaver, F. (2005), The inequality of social capital and the reproduction of chronic poverty. *World Development* 33 (6): 893- 906.

Cohen, A.P. (1985), *The Symbolic Construction of Community,* London: Tavistock or Routledge.

Coleman, J. (1988), Social capital in the creation of human capital. *American Journal of Sociology* 94 (Supplement): S95- S120.

Coleman, J. (1990), *Foundations of Social Theory*. Cambridge, Mass: Harvard University Press.

Corbett, E.L., R.W. Steketee, F.O. ter Kuile, A.S Latif, A. Kamali & P.J. Hayes (2001), AIDS in Africa and the control of other infectious diseases. *Lancet* 359: 2177-2187.

Costa, D.L. & M.E. Kahn (2002), Civic engagement and community heterogeneity. An ecomonist perspective. *Perspectives on Politics* 1:103-111.

Creighton, C. (1995), Kinship in the urban setting in Tanzania. In: C. Creighton & C. K. Omari (Eds.) *Gender, Family and Work in Tanzania*. Aldershot, Burlington USA, Singapore and Sydney: Ashgate, pp 67-125.

Crowe, G. (1989), The use of the concept 'strategy' in recent sociological literature. *Sociology* 23: 1-24.

Davies, S. (1993), Are coping strategies a cop out? *IDS Bulletin* 24:60-72.

Davies, S. (1996), *Adaptable Livelihoods: Coping with Food Insecurity in the Malian Sahel*, New York, London: Macmillan Press.

Davies, S., M. Schneide, G. Papholo & D. Everatt (1997), *Guidelines for developing a workplace policy and programme on HIV/AIDS and STDs*. Pretoria, Southern Africa Department of Health.

De Haan, L. (2000), Globalisation, localization and sustainable livelihood. Sociologia Ruralis 40(3): 339-365.

De Waal, A. (1989), *Famine that kills: Darfur Sudan 1984-1985*. Oxford: Clarenddon Press.

De Waal, A. & A. Whiteside (2003), New Variant Famine: AIDS and Food Crisis in Southern Africa. *The Lancet* 362(9391): 1234-1237.

De Waal, A. & J. Tumushabe (2003), *HIV/AIDS and Food Security in Africa*. A report for Department for International Development, London: DFID.

De Waal, A. (2003), How will HIV/AIDS transform African Governance? *African Affairs* 102: 1-23.

Decosas, J. (2002), *The social ecology of AIDS in Africa*. UNRISD project HIV/AIDS and Development: Geneva.

Desmond, C., K. Michael & J. Gow (2000), *The hidden battle: HIV/AIDS in the family and community*. University of Natal, Durban: Health Economics and HIV/AIDS Research Division (HEARD).

Dercon, S. (2005), Vulnerability: a micro perspective. A paper presented at the Annual Bank Conference on Development Economics (ABCDE) for Europe. World Bank conference May 2005, Amsterdam.

Devereux, S. (2001), Livelihood insecurity and social protection: A re-emerging issue in Rural Development. *Development Policy Review* 19(4): 507-519.

Devereux, S. (1993), *Theories of Famine*. London: Harvester Wheatsheaf.

DFID (2000), *Sustainable livelihoods guidance sheets*. Available on line at: http//www.livelihoods.org/info/info-guidance sheets.html. (Accessed on 7/12/ 2005).

Dhesi, A.S. (2000), Social capital and community development. *Community Development Journal* 35(3): 199-214.

DiPasquale, D. & E. Glaeser (1999), Incentives and social capital: are homeowners better citizens. *Journal of Urban Economics* 45(2):354-384.

Dikito-Wachtmeister, M.S. (2001), *Empowering women to achieve Food Security – Social capital*. International Food Policy Research Institute (IFPRI) 2020 Focus 6, Brief 9. Washington DC: IFPRI.

Donahue, J., K. Kubbucho & S. Osinde (2001) Responding to a silent economic crisis among microfinance clients in Kenya and Uganda. Nairobi, Kenya: Microsave. www.microsave.com (Accessed on 25/06/07).

Drinkwater, M., M. McEwan & F. Samuels (2006), *Understanding HIV/AIDS and livelihoods: The contribution of longitudinal data and cluster analysis*. Overseas Development Institute Briefing paper 8. London: ODI.

Drinkwater, M. (2003), HIV/AIDS and agrarian change in Southern Africa. Presentation for the United Nations Regional Inter-Agency Coordination and Support Office Technical Consultation on Vulnerability in the light of an HIV/AIDS pandemic. 9-11 September 2003, Johannesburg, South Africa.

Durlauf, S.N. & M. Fafchamps (2004), Empirical studies of social capital. *NBER Working paper 10485* http://www.nber.org/papers/w10485 (Accessed on 24/03/06: 1705).

Eakin, H. (2005), Institutional change, climate risk, and rural vulnerability: Cases from Central Mexico. *World Development* 33(11):1923-1938

Ellis, F. (1998), Household livelihood strategies and rural livelihood diversification. *Journal of Development Studies* 35(1): 1-38.

Ellis, F. (2000), *Rural livelihoods and Diversity in Developing Countries*. Oxford: Oxford University Press.

Economic and Social Research Foundation (2003) *The economic and social impacts of HIV/AIDS in Tanzania*. Final Report. Dar es salaam: ESRF.

Economic and Social Research Foundation (2005) *The impacts of HIV/AIDS on agriculture: The case of Kilombero and Ulanga District*. Areport submitted to EZCORE, Ilonga Kilosa: ESRF.

Food and Agriculture Organization (1997), *Report of the World Food Summit, 13-17 November 1996*. Rome: FAO

Food and Agriculture Organization (1995), *Feminization of Agriculture*. Rome: FAO.

Fapohunda, E.P. (1988), The non-pooling household, a challenge to theory. In: B. Dwyer, (Ed.) *A home divided; women and income in the Third World*. Stanford: University Press, pp. 143-154.

Farrington, J., D. Carney, C. Ashley & C. Turton (1999), *Sustainable livelihood in practice: early application of concepts in rural areas*. London: ODI Natural Resource Perspective 42.

Field, A. (2005), Discovering Statistics using SPSS. London, Thousand Oaks, New Delhi: SAGE Publications. (Second edition).

Finch, J. & J. Mason (1993), *Negotiating Family Responsibilities*. London and New York: Tavistock/ Routledge.

Finch, J. (1987), Family obligations and the life course. In: A. Bryman, B. Bytheway, P. Allatt, & T. Keil (Eds.) *Rethinking the Life Cycle*. Hampshire and London: The Macmillan Press, pp. 234-267.

Fine, B. (2001), *Social Capital versus Social theory*. London and New York: Routledge.

Food Consumption and Nutrition Division (FCND) (1999), *Technical guide for operationalizing household food security in development project*. Washington DC: International Food Policy Research Institute.

Foster, G. (2005), Under the radar: community safety-nets for children affected by HIV/AIDS in poor households in Sub-Saharan Africa. A paper prepared for the United Nations Research Institute for Social Development Training and Research Support Centre programme on Community Responses to HIV and AIDS. Geneva: UNRISD.

Frankenberger, T. & M. McCaston (1998), The household livelihood security concept. *Food and Nutrition and Agriculture* 22:30-35.

Fukuyama, F. (1995), *Trust: Social Values and the Creation of Prosperity*. New York: Free Press.

Gillespie, S. (2006), AIDS, Poverty, and Hunger: An Overview. In: S. Gillespie (Ed.) *AIDS, Poverty, and Hunger: Challenges and Responses*. Highlights of the International Conference on HIV/AIDS and Food and Nutrition Security, April 14-16, 2005, Durban, South Africa. Washington, DC: International Food Policy Research Institute (IFPRI).

Gillespie, S. & S. Kadiyala (2005), HIV/AIDS and Food and Nutrition Security: From Evidence to Action. *Food Policy Review 7*. Washington, DC: International Food Policy Research Institute (IFPRI).

Gillespie, S. & M. Loevinsohn (2003), Applying an HIV/AIDS lens to agricultural policy. *RENEWAL Working Paper No.2*. Washington and The Hague: International Food Policy Research Institute (IFPRI)/International Service for National Agricultural Research (ISNAR).

Gillian, P. (1996), *Women in the times of AIDS*. Maryknoll, New York: Orbis Books.

Gillies, P. (1998), Effectiveness of alliances and partnership for health promotion. *Health Promotion International* 13:1-21.

Glaeser, E.D., D. Laibson & B. Sacerdote (2000), The economic approach to social capital. *NBER Working Paper 7728*. Cambridge Massachusetts: National Bureau of Economic Research, Inc.

Godquin, M. & A. Quisumbing (2005), Groups, networks and social capital in rural Philippine Communities. A paper presented in International Research group on Gender and collective action 17-21 October 2005 Chiang Mai, Thailand.

Golooba-Mutebi, F. (2003), Witchcraft and social relations in a South African village: implications for development policy and practice. Development Research Centre's Crisis States Programme *Seminar series 3.* London School of Economics and Political Science.

Golooba-Mutebi, F. (2005), Witchcraft, social cohesion and participation in a South African village. *Development and Change* 36(5):937-958.

Green, M. (2005), Discourses on inequality. Poverty, public bads and entrenching witchcraft in post-adjustment Tanzania. *Anthropological Theory* 5(3): 247-266

Green, M. (2000), Public reforms and privatization of poverty: Some institutional determinants of healing seeking behaviours in Southern Tanzania. *Culture, Medicine and Psychiatry* 24:403-430.

Green, M. (1993), *The construction of religion and the pertuation of tradition among the Pogoro Catholics, Southern Tanzania.* Unpublished PhD. Thesis, London School of Economics and Political Science.

Green, M. (1994), Shaving witchcraft in Ulanga. In: R. Abrahams (Ed.) *Witchcraft in Contemporary Tanzania.* University of Cambridge UK: African Studies Centre, pp. 23-46.

Groat, M. (1997), The informal organization: Ride the headless monster. *Management Accounting 75*(4): 40-42.

Grootaert, C., G.T. Oh, & A. Swamy (1999), The local level institutions study: Social capital and development outcomes in Burkina Faso. Local Level Institutions *Working Paper No.7.* Washington DC: World Bank.

Grootaert, C. & T. van Bastelaer (2002), Social capital: From definition to measurement. In: C. Grootaert & T. van Bastelaer (Eds.) *Understanding and measuring social capital: a multidisciplinary tool for practioners.* Washington DC: World Bank, pp.1-16.

Guyer, J. & P. Peters (1988), Conceptualizing the household: Introduction. *Development and change* 18 (2): 197-214.

Guyer, J. (1980), Household budgets and women's incomes. *Working Paper 28.* Boston University, Boston, Mass: African Studies Center.

Haddad, L & S. Gillespie (2001), Effective food and nutritional policy responses to HIV/AIDS. What we know and what we need to know. *Journal of international Development* 13:487-511.

Hanson, S. (2000), Health sector reforms and STD/AIDS control in resource poor setting. The case of Tanzania. *International Journal of Health planning and management* 15:341-360.

Harris, C.C. (1990), *Kinship.* Buckingham: Open University Press.

Harris, J. (2001), Social capital and the construction of civil society in rural areas. *Working paper 01-16.* London: London School of Economics and Political Science.

Hartl, M. (2003), *Rural women's access to land and property in selected countries. Analysis based on initial and periodic reports to the Committee on the Elimination of Discrimination against Women (1997-2003).* Rome: FAO/IFAD/International Land Coalition.

Hawton, M., G. Hughes & J. Percy-Smith (1999), *Community Profiling-Auditing Social Needs.* Buckingham: Open University Press.

Hearn, J. (2000), Aiding democracy? Donors and civil society in South Africa. *Third World Quarterly,* 21(5): 815-830

Heuveline, P. (2004), Impacts of HIV epidemic on population and household structure: the dynamics and evidence to date. *AIDS* 18 (Supplement 2):45-53.

Howard, M.C. (1986), *Contemporary Cultural Anthropology*. Boston, Toronto: Little Brown and Company, pp. 183-203.

Hussein A.K & P.G. Mujinja (1997), Impact of user charge on government health facilities in Tanzania. *East African Medical journal* 74(12): 751-57.

Hutchful, E. (1996), The civil society debate in Africa. *International Journal* 51(1):54-77.

International Center for Research on Women (ICRW) (2002), Understanding HIV-related stigma and resulting discrimination in Sub-Saharan Africa. Emerging themes from early data collection in Ethiopia, Tanzania and Zambia. *Research update*. Washington DC: ICRW.

International Center for Research on Women (2003), *Disentangling HIV and AIDS stigma in Ethiopia, Tanzania and Zambia*. Washington DC: ICRW.

International Fund for Agricultural Development (IFAD) (1998), *Food security, poverty and women: Lessons from Rural Asia, Part 1*. Rome: IFAD/TAD.

Jamil, I. & R. Muriisa (2004), Building social capital in Uganda: The role of NGOs in mitigating HIV/AIDS challenges. A paper presented at the International Conference organized by the International Society for Third Sector Research (ISTR) 11-14 July 2004, Toronto.

Jutting, J. (1999), Strengthening social security systems in rural areas of developing countries. Zentrum fur Entwicklungsforschung Center for Development Research *Discussion paper on Development Policy*: University of Bonn, Germany.

Kaag, M., R. van Berkel, J. Brons, M. de Bruijn, H. van Dijk, L. de Haan, G. Nooteboom & A. Zoomers (2004), Ways forward in livelihood research. In: D. Kalb, W. Pansters & H. Siebers (Eds.) *Globalization and Development: Themes and concepts in current research*. Dordrecht, Boston, London Kluwer Academic Publishers, pp. 49-74.

Kabeer, N. (1991), Gender, production and well being: Rethinking the household economy. Institute of Development Studies *Discussion paper 288*. Brighton: IDS.

Kabeer, N. (1994), *Reversed Realities: Gender, Hierarchies in Development Thought*. London, New York: Verso.

Kabeer, N. (2003), *Gender Mainstreaming in Poverty Eradication and the Millennium Development Goals*. A handbook for policy-makers and other stakeholders. Commonwealth Secretariat. Ottawa, Cairo, Dakar, Montevideo, Nairobi, New Delhi, Singapore: International Development Research Centre

Kakuru, D.M. (2006), *The combat for gender equality in education. Rural livelihood pathways in the context of HIV/AIDS*. African women leaders in agriculture and the environment (AWLAE) series No. 4. Wageningen: Wageningen Academic Publishers.

Kashuliza, A.K. & E.R. Mbiha (1995), Structural adjustment and the performance of the agricultural sector in Tanzania, 1980-1990. In: P. G. Forster & S. Maghimbi (Eds.) *Tanzanian Peasantry: Further Studies*, Aldershot and Brookfield VT: Avebury, pp. 51-77.

Katz, E. (1997), The intra-household economics of voice and exit. *Feminist Economics* 3(3): 25-46.

Kavishe, F.P & S.S Mushi (1993), Nutrition-relevant actions in Tanzania. Tanzania Food and Nutrition Centre, Case study for the 15th Congress of the International Union of Nutritional Science, September 26th to October 1st 1993. Adelaide.

Kawachi, I. & L. Berkman (2000), Social cohesion, social capital and health. In: L. Berkman & I. Kawachi (Eds.) *Social Epidemiology*. Oxford: Oxford University Press, pp. 174-190.

Kertzer, D.I. (1986). A life course approach to co-residence. In: D.I. Kertzer (Ed.) *Family Relations in Life Course Perspective*. Current Perspectives on Aging and the Life Cycle, vol. 2. Greenwich: JAI Press, pp.1-22.

Kikula, I.S., E.Z. Mnzava & C. Mungóngó (2003), Shortcomings of the Linkages between Environmental Conservation Initiatives and Poverty Allevation in Tanzania. *Research Report no 03.2.* Dar es Salaam: Research on Poverty Alleviation (REPOA)

Kilombero District Development Plans (2003), Morogoro, Tanzania. (Unpublished report).

Kilombero District HIV/AIDS Report (2004), Morogoro, Tanzania. (Unpublished report).

Kironde, J.M.L. (2004), *Current changes in customary/traditional land delivery systems in sub-Saharan African cities: The case of Dar es Salaam city*. 2005. www.ucl.ac.uk/dpu/research/housing/Tanzania%20Final.pdf (accessed on 29/01/2007: 1445)

Knack, S. & P. Keefer (1997), Does social capital have an economic payoff? A cross-country investigation. *Quarterly Journal of Economics* 112 (4):1251-1288.

Koda, B.O. (1995), The economic organization of the household in contemporary Tanzania. In: C. Creighton & C.K. Omary (Eds.) *Gender, Family and Household in Tanzania*. Aldershot, Brookfield USA, Singapore, Sydney: Avebury, pp. 139-155.

Koopman, J. (1991), Neoclassical household models and modes of household production: problems in the analysis of African Agricultural households. *Review of radical political economies* 23(3&4): 148-173.

Lazaro, E.A. (1996) *Women in the Household Economy: The Case of Agricultural Plantations in Morogoro Region, Tanzania.* Unpublished PhD. thesis, Sokoine University of Agriculture.

Letki, N. (2005), *Does diversity erode social cohesion? Social capital and race in British Neighbourhood.* www.nuffield.ox.ac.uk/Politics/Papers/2005/NLetki-diversity social capital.pdf (Accessed on 24/03/06: 1645)

Liviga, A.J. & R.D.K Mekacha (1998), *Youth Migration and Poverty Alleviation: A case study of Petty traders (Wamachinga) in Dar es Salaam.* Dar es Salaam: Research on Poverty Alleviation (REPOA).

Loevinsohn, M. & S. Gillespie (2003), HIV/AIDS, food security and rural livelihoods: Understanding and responding. Regional Network on HIV/AIDS, Rural Livelihoods and Food Security *Working paper no. 2*, Washington DC: RENEWAL.

Lowndes, V. (2000), Women and social capital: a comment on Hall's 'Social Capital in Britain'. *British Journal of Political Science* 30(3): 533-540.

Lowndes, V. (2003), Getting on or getting by? Women, social capital and political participation. *British Journal of Politics and International Relations* 6: 45-64.

Lundberg, M., M. Over & P. Mujinja (2000), Sources of financial assistance for households suffering an adult death in Kagera, Tanzania. *The South African Journal of Economics* 68 (5): 139.

Luxton, M. (1997), The UN, women and the household labour: measuring and valuing unpaid work. *Women's Studies International Forum* 20 (3): 431-439.

Lwihula, G. (1999), Coping with AIDS Pandemic: The experience of peasant communities of Kagera Region, Tanzania. In: G. Mutangadura, H. Jackson & D. Mukurazita (Eds.). *AIDS and African Smallholder Agriculture.* SAfAIDS. Harare, Zimbabwe: MG Printers, pp. 153-159.

Lyon, F. (2000), Trust, networks and norms: The creation of social capital in Agricultural economies in Ghana. *World Development* 28(4): 663-681.

Mackay, V. (2003), *Best practices in HIV/AIDS prevention in the informal sector.* Geneva, Inter-regional tripartite meeting on best practices in workplace policies and programmes on HIV/AIDS. Available at http://www.ilo.org/public/english /protection /trav/aids/publ/ informalecoprev.pdf (Accessed on 30/08/2006: 1535).

Madembo, R.C. (1997), The role of saving and credits schemes in meeting social security needs of communal farmers. In: E. Kaseke (Ed.) *Social Security systems in Rural Zimbabwe,* Harare: Friedrich Ebert Stiftung.

Makundi, E.A., J. Nyoni & P. Nanda (2005), The implications of health sector reforms on reproductive health services. The case of Bukoba District - Kagera Region, Tanzania study. *Center for Health and Gender Equity working Paper.* Takoma Park, MD, USA: Center for Health and Gender Equity.

Maluccio, J., L. Haddad & J. May (2000), Social capital and households welfare in South Africa. *Journal of Development studies,* 36 (6): 54-81.

Mapolu, H. (1990) Tanzania: Imperialism, the state of peasantry in African Agriculture: In: A. A. Hamid & B. F. Tchuigona (Eds.) *The Critical Choices.* Tokyo, London and New Jersey: United University Press, pp. 138-148.

Maxwell, S. (2001), The evolution of thinking about food security. In: S. Devereux & S. Maxwell (Eds.) *Food Security in Sub-Saharan Africa.* IDS Brighton: ITDG Publishing, pp. 13-27.

Maxwell, J. (1997), *Social cohesion: a test for political process.* (Speech in a symposium for new members of the Canadian Parliament at Queen's school of policy studies) http://www.cprn.com/jmaxwell/files/spsct_e.htm, Toronto. (Accessed on 28/09/2003: 1732).

Maxwell, S. (1996), Food security: a postmodern perspective. *Food Policy,* 21 (2) 155-170.

Maxwell, S. & T. Frankenberger (1992), *Household Food Security: Concepts, Indicators, Measurement:* A Technical Review. New York, Rome: UNICEF and IFAD.

May, T. (1997), Interviewing : Methods and process. In: T. May (Ed.) *Social Research: Issues, Methods and Process.* Buckingham and Philadephia: Open University Press, pp. 109-131.

Mayoux, L. (2001), Tackling the downside: social capital, women's empowerment and micro-finance in Cameroon. *Development and change* 32: 435- 464.

Mbilinyi, M. (1997), *The end of smallholder farming?: Gender and Structural Adjustment.* Electronic publication from University of Dar es salaam, Tanzania. (Accessed on 22/04/06 at 1343).

McCracken, M. (1998), Social cohesion and macroeconomics performance. A paper presented at the state of living standards and the quality of life Conference 30-31 October 1998 Ottawa, Ontario/Canada: Centre for the study of living standards (CSLS).

McCrone, D. (1994), Getting by and making out. In: M. Anderson, F. Bechhofer & J. Gershuny (Eds.) *The social and Political economy of the Household.* Oxford: Oxford University Press, pp. 68-99.

Mesaki, S. (1994), Witch-killing in Sukumaland. In: R. Abrahams (Ed.) *Witchcraft in Contemporary Tanzania.* University of Cambridge: African Studies Center, pp. 47-60.

Midgley, J. (1995), *Social Development: The Developmental Perspective in Social Welfare.* London: Sage Publication.

Mingione, E. (1987), Urban survival strategies, family structure and informal practices. In: M.P. Smith & J.R. Foggin (Eds.) *The Capitalist City: Global Restructuring and Community Politics.* Oxford: Basil Blackwood Ltd, pp. 297-322.

Ministry of Health (1996), *Health Sector Reform Plan of Action 1996-1999.* Dar es salaam, Tanzania.

Ministry of Health (1997), *Report of Health Sector Reform Program of Work 1998/99-2000/2001.* Draft. Dar es Salaam, Tanzania.

Ministry of Health (1999), Health Sector plan of Action July 1999 - June 2000. Dar es Salaam.

Mkamba Village report (2003), Kilombero District, Morogoro (Unpublished report).

Moerbeek, H. (2001), *Friends and foes in the occupational career. The influence of sweet and sour social capital on the labout market.* Unpublished PhD. thesis Nijmegen University.

Mohga, K.S. (2002), Gender, poverty, and intergenerational vulnerability to HIV/AIDS. *Gender and Development Journal* 10(3): 63- 70.

Molyneux, M. (2002), Gender and the silence of social capital: lessons from Latin America. *Development and change* 33(2): 167-188.

Morduch, J. (1999), Between the state and the market: can informal insurance patch the safety net? *World Bank Research Observer* 14 (2):187-207.

Moser, C. (1993), *Gender Planning and Development: Theory, Practice and Training.* London: Routledge.

Moser, C. (1996), *Confronting crisis: A comparative study of household responses to poverty and vulnerability in four poor urban communities.* Environmentally Sustainable Development Studies and Monographs Series No. 8. Washington DC: The World Bank.

Moser, C. (1998), Gender planning in the Third World: meeting practical and strategic gender needs. *World Development* 30 (3): 435- 464.

Mtika, M.M. (2001), AIDS epidemic in Malawi and its threat to household food security. *Human Organization* 60 (2): 178-188.

Mtshali, S.M. (2002), *Household livelihood security in rural KwaZulu Natal, South Africa.* PhD Thesis Wageningen University.

Mubyazi G.M, J.J. Massaga, K.J. Njunwa, K.Y. Mdira, F.M. Salum, M.S. Alilio & M.L. Kamugisha (2000), Health financing policy in Tanzania: Payment mechanism for poor vulnerable groups in Korogwe District. *Small Applied Research Report 13.* Bethasda MD: Partnership for Health Reforms Project, Abt Associates Inc.

Muela, S.H., A.K. Mushi & J.M. Ribera (2000), The paradox of the cost and affordability of traditional and government health services in Tanzania. *Health Policy and Planning* 15: 296-302.

Müller, T. (2005), *HIV/AIDS, gender and rural livelihoods in sub-Saharan Africa. An overview and annotated bibliography*. Wageningen: Wageningen Academic Publishers.

Müller, T. (2004a), *HIV/AIDS and agriculture in sub-Saharan Africa. Impact on farming systems, Agri-cultural practices and rural livelihoods – an overview and annotated bibliography* Wageningen: Wageningen Academic Publishers.

Müller, T. (2004b), Moving beyond the household. Some comments on the theoretical underpinnings of Anke Niehof's 'micro-ecological' approach to health. *Medische Antropologie* 16 (2): 269-271.

Munishi, G. (2003), Intervening to address constraints through health sector reforms in Tanzania: some gains and the unfinished business. *Journal of Iinternational Development* 15:115-131.

Murphy, M. (1987), Measuring the life cycle: concepts, data and Methods. In: A. Bryman, B. Bytheway, P. Allatt, & T. Keil (Eds.) *Rethinking theLlife Cycle*. Hampshire and London: Macmillan Press, pp. 30-52.

Murray, U. (2005), Promoting gender-sensitive entrepreneurship via microfinance institutions. Rome, Paper presented at FAO Headquarters on International Women's Day. Available at http://www.fao.org/sd/dim_pe1/pe1_050401_en.htm (Accessed on 29/8/06: 1115).

Mutangadura G., D. Mukurazita & H. Jackson (1999), *A review of household and community responses to the HIV/AIDS in rural areas of sub-Sahara Africa.* UNAIDS Best Practice Paper. Geneva: UNAIDS.

Mwakalobo, A. (2003), *Implications of HIV/AIDS on rural livelihoods in Tanzania: The case of Rungwe District*. Morogoro, Tanzania: Development Studies Institute, Sokoine University of Agriculture.

Mwalimu, U.A. (2004), Patterns, policy and legal issues on international labour Migration in Tanzania. *Economic and Social Research Foundation Globalization working paper Series no.3.* Dar es Salaam: ESRF.

Mwisongo A., L. Mboera, M. Alilio, W. Kisoka, M. Kamugisha, P. Mutalemwa, C. Kabali, M. Malecela & A. Kitua (2000), *Situational analysis of 37 Districts for phase one of health sector reforms.* Dar es Salaam: National Institute for Medical Research and Ministry of Health.

Mwisongo, A., E. Makundi, L. Kisinza & L.E Mborea (2000), *Situational analysis of 45 councils under phase II of the joint health Sector/Local Government reforms.* Dar es Salaam: National Institute for Medical Research and Ministry of Health.

Nanda, P. (2000), Health sector reforms in Zambia: implications for reproductive health and rights. *Center for Health and Gender Equity Working paper*. Tacoma Park, MD: Center for Health and Gender Equity.

Nanda, P. (2002), Gender dimension of user fees: Implications for women's utilization of Health care. *Reproductive Health Matters* 10(20): 127-128.

Narayan, D. (1997), *Voices of the poor: poverty and social capital in Tanzania.* Environmentally and Socially Sustainable Development Studies and Monographs Series, No. 20. Washington DC: World Bank.

Narayan, D. & L. Prichett (1999), Cents and sociability: household income and social capital in rural Tanzania. *Economic development and Cultural changes* 47(4): 871-97.

Ngom, P. & S. Clark (2003), Adult mortality in the era of HIV/AIDS: Sub-Saharan Africa. A paper presented in a workshop on HIV/AIDS and adult mortality in developing countries 8-13 September 2003, New York.

Niehof, A. (1999), *Household, Family and Nutrition research: Writing a Proposal*. Wageninge H & C Publication series 1, Wageningen University.

Niehof, A. (2002), The household production of care. In: C. Buijn, P. Groot-Marcus, M. van der Linden, L.P.A. Steenbekkers, P.M.J. Terpstra (Eds.) *Changes at the other end of the chain: everyday consumption in a multidisciplinary perspective*. The Netherlands: Shaker Publishing, pp. 179-188.

Niehof, A. (2003a), Why kinship, what is it and how to do it? Unpublished lecture notes. Wageningen University.

Niehof, A. (2003b), Gendered dynamics of food security at the household level. In: U. Karim (Ed.) *No security without food security-No food security without gender equality*. Association of World Council of Churches Related Development Organisations in Europe (APRODEV) GOOD Conference Report, Brussels: APRODEV, pp. 60- 68.

Niehof, A. (2004a), The significance of diversification for rural livelihoods systems. *Food Policy* 29: 321-338.

Niehof, A. (2004b), A micro-ecological approach to home care for AIDS patients. *Medische Antropologie* 16 (2):245-265.

Niehof, A. (2004c) Why should households care? *Medische Antropologie* 16(2): 282-289.

Niehof, A. & L. Price (2001), *Rural livelihood systems: A conceptual framework*. Wageningen-UPWARD Series on Rural Livelihoods No. 1. Wageningen: WU-UPWARD.

Nkurunziza, E. & C. Rakodi (2005), Urban families under pressure: conceptual and methodological issues in the study of poverty, HIV/AIDS and livelihood strategies. *Urban household livelihoods and HIV/AIDS Working Paper 1*. University of Birmingham: International Development Department.

Nnko, S, B. Chiduo, F. Wilson, W. Msuta & G. Mwaluko (2000), Tanzania: AIDS Care - learning from experience. *Review of African Political Economy* 86: 547-557.

Nooteboom, G. (2003) *A matter of style, social security and livelihood in upland East Java*. PhD. thesis, Nijmegen University.

North, D. (1990), *Institutions, Institutional Change, and Economic Performance*. New York: Cambridge University Press.

O'Laughlin, B. (1995), Myth of the African family in the world Development. In: D. Bryceson (Ed.) *Women Wielding the Hoe: Lessons from rural Africa for Feminist Theory and Development Practice*. Washington DC: Berg Publishers Oxford, pp. 63-91.

Omari, C.K. (1995), Decision making and the household: Case study from Tanzania. In: C. Creighton & C.K. Omari (Eds.) *Gender, Family and Household in Tanzania*. Aldershot, Brookfield USA, Singapore, Sydney: Avebury, pp. 203-220.

Omosa, M. (1998), *Re-conceptualising food security; interlocking strategies, unfolding choices and rural livelihoods in Kisii District, Kenya*. PhD. Thesis, Wageningen Univeristy.

Onyx, J. & R. Leonard (2002), The relationship between formal and informal volunteering: A social capital framework. A paper presented at the ISTR Fifth International Conference on Transforming Civil Society, Citizenship and Governance: The Third Sector in an Era of Global (Dis)Order, July 7-10, 2002, Cape Town, South Africa.

Oorschot, W. & W. Arts (2004), The social capital of European welfare states. The crowding out hypothesis revisited. A paper presented at the 2nd Annual ESPAnet Conference, Meeting the Needs of a New Europe, 9-11 September 2004, Oxford UK.

Orvis, S. (2001), Civil society in Africa or African civil society? *Journal of Asian & African Studies* 36(1): 17-39.

Ostrom, E. (1999), Social capital: a fad or a fundamental concept. In: P. Dasgupta & I. Serageld (Eds.) *Social Capital: A Multifaceted Perspective* Washington DC: World Bank, pp. 172-214.

Ottosson, C. (1999), *Capitalism and Kinship in Africa*. Uppsala University: Institution of National Economics.

Pennartz, P. & A. Niehof (1999), *The Domestic Domain: Chances Choices and Strategies of Family Households*. Aldershot, Burlington USA, Singapore, Sydney: Ashgate.

Perlas, N. (2000), *Shaping Globalization, Civil Society, Cultural Power and Threefolding*. South Africa: The Novalis Press.

Picciotto, S. (1998), Linkages in international investment regulation: the antinomies of the draft multilateral agreement on investment. *University of Pennsylvania Journal of International Economic Law,*19.

Platteau, J.P. (1991), Traditional systems of social security and hunger insurance: past achievement and modern challenges. In: E. Ahmad, J. Dreze, J. Hills, & A. Sen (Eds.) *Social security in Developing countries*. Oxford: Clarendon Press, pp. 112-170.

Portes, A. (1998), Social Capital: its origins and applications in modern sociology. *Annual Review of Sociology* 22: 1-24.

Portes A. & J. Sensenbrenner (1993), Embeddedness and immigration: notes on the social determinants of economic action. *American Journal of Sociology* 98: 1320-1350.,

Portes, A. & Landolt, P. (1996), The downside of social capital. *The American Prospects*. 26: 18-22.

Price, L. & M. Brouns (1999), *Science by and for women in developing countries*. The Hague: UNESCO Network on Women and Technology, Ministry of Foreign Affairs, The Hague.

Putnam, R. (1993), *Making Democracy Work: Civic Traditions in Modern Italy*. Princeton: Princeton University Press.

Putnam, R. (2000), *Bowling Alone: The Collapse and Revival of American Community*. New York: Simon and Schuster.

Putnam, R. (2007), *E Pluribus Unum*: Diversity and community in the twenty-first century. The 2006 Johan Skytte Prize Lecture. *Scandinavian Political Studies* 30(2): 137-174.

Putzel, J. (1997), Accounting for the 'dark side' of social capital: reading Robert Putnam on democracy. *Journal of international Development* 9 (7): 939-949.

Radstake, M. (2000), *Secrecy and ambiguity. Home care for people living with HIV/AIDS in Ghana*. African Studies Centre research report 59/2000, Leiden: African Studies Centre.

Rakodi, C. (1999), A capital asset framework for analyzing household livelihood strategies: implication for policy review. *Development Policy Review* 17: 315-342.

Rankin, C.N. (2002), Social capital, microfinance and the politics of development. *Feminist Economics* 8(1): 1-24.

Riet, H., A.P. den Hartog, A.M. Mwangi, R.K.N. Mwadime, D.W.J. Foeken & W.A. van Staveren (2001), The role of street foods in the dietary pattern of two low-income groups in Nairobi. *European Journal of Clinical Nutrition* 55: 562-570.

Robb, C. (1998), Social aspects of the East Asian financial crisis: perceptions of poor communities. Paper presented at the East Asia Crisis workshop at the Institute of Development Studies, University of Sussex UK. http:// www.ids.ac.uk/ids/ research/ robb.pdf (Accessed on 27/02/04: 1050).

Rose, R. (1999) What does social capital add to individual welfare? An imperial analysis of Russia. World Bank social capital initiative *Working paper no. 15*. Washington DC: World Bank.

Rose, R. (1997), *Measures of social capital in African surveys*. World Bank social capital initiative. Washington DC: World Bank.

Rotheram-Borus, M.J., D. Flannery & P. Lester (2005), Families living with HIV. *AIDS Care* 17 (8): 978-987.

Rudd, M.A. (2000), Live long and prosper: collective action, social capital and social Vision. *Ecological Economics* 34 (234): 131-144.

Rudie, I. (1995), The significance of 'eating': cooperation, support and reputation in Lelantan Malay households. In: W. Karim (Ed.) *'Male' and 'Female' in Developing Southeast Asia*. Oxford, Washington: Berg Publishers, pp. 227-245.

Rugalema, G. (1999a), *Adult mortality as entitlement failure: AIDS and the crisis of rural livelihoods in a Tanzanian village*. PhD thesis, Institute of Social Studies, Den Haag.

Rugalema, G. (1999b), It is not only the loss of labour: HIV/AIDS, loss of household assets and household livelihood in Bukoba District, Tanzania. In: G. Mutangadura, H. Jackson & D. Mukurazita (Eds.) *AIDS and African Smallholder Agriculture*. Harare, Zimbabwe: MG Printers. Southern Africa HIV and AIDS Information Dissemination Service (SAFAIDS) pp. 41-52.

Rugalema, G. (2000), Coping or struggling? A journey into the impacts of HIV/AIDS in Southern Africa. *Review of African Political Economy* 86: 537-545.

Russell, S (2005), Illuminating cases: understanding the economic burden of illness through case study household research. *Health Policy and Planning* 20(55): 277-289.

Southern African Development Community (SADC) (2003) *Towards Identifying Impacts of HIV/ AIDS on Food Insecurity in Southern Africa and Implications for Response. Findings from Malawi, Zambia and Zimbabwe*. Harare, Zimbabwe: FANR Vulnerability assessment Committee.

Sabatini, F. (2005), Social capital as social networks. A new framework for measurement. Roma: Dipartimento di Economia Pubblica, *Working paper 83*. Universita' Degli Studi di Roma'la Sapienza'

Sahn, D.E., S.D. Young & G. Genicot (2003), Health care demands in rural Tanzania. *Oxford Bulletin of Economics and Statistics* 65(2): 241-259.

Sauerborn R., A. Adams & M. Hien (1996), Household strategies to cope with the economic costs of illness. *Social Science and Medicine* 43(11): 291-301.

Schellenberg, J., C. Victoria, A. Mushi, D. de Savingy, D. Schellenberg, H. Mshiinnda & J. Bryce (2003), Inequalities among very poor: health care for children in rural Southern Tanzania. *The Lancet* 361(9357): 561-566.

Scott, J.C. (1976), *The Moral Economy of the Peasant: Rebellion and Subsistence in Southeast Asia.* New Haven: Yale University Press.

Scrimshaw, S.C.M. (1990), Combining quantitative and qualitative methods in the study of intra-household resource allocation. In: B. L. Rogers & N. P. Schlossman (Eds.) *Intra-Household Resource Allocation: Issues and Methods for Development Policy and Planning.* Tokyo: United Nations University Press, pp. 86-98.

Sen, A. (1981), *Poverty and Famines: An Essay on Entitlement and Deprivation.* Oxford: Clarendon Press.

Sen, A. (1990), Gender and Cooperative conflicts. In: I. Tinker (Ed.) *Persistent Inequalities: Women and World Development.* New York, Oxford: Oxford University Press, pp. 124-149.

Sen, B. (2002), Risks, vulnerability and poverty in Bangladesh: issues and evidence: variation on a theme. www.bids.org/sen2002.doc. (Accessed on 11/12/2005:1935).

Seandaro, A.M. (1991), Socialist Policy and land tenure in Tanzania. In: J. Hartmann (Ed.) Re thinking of Arusha Declaration. Copenhagen: Center for Development Research, pp. 262-269.

Sharon, L.L. (1999), Sampling: Design and Analysis. Pacific Grove, Albany, Belmont, Bonn: Duxburg Press.

Silvey, R. & R. Elmhirst (2003), Engendering social capital: women workers and rural-urban networks in Indonesia's crisis. *World Development* 31(5): 865-879.

Simon, V., D.D. Ho & Q. Abdool-Karim (2006), HIV/AIDS epidemiology, pathogenesis, prevention, and treatment. *The Lancet* 368: 489-504.

Skarstein, R. (2005), Economic liberalization and smallholder productivity in Tanzania. From promised to real failure, 1985-1998. *Journal of Agrarian Change* 5(3): 334-365.

Stillwaggon, E. (2006), *AIDS and the ecology of Poverty.* Oxford and New York: Oxford University Press.

Stone, W. (2001), Measuring social capital: Towards a theoretically informed measurement framework for researching social capital in family and community life. Australian Institute of Family Studies, *Research Paper No. 24.* Melbourne: Australian Institute of Family Studies.

Stone, W. & J. Hughes (2001), The nature and distribution of social capital: initial findings of the Families, Social capital and Citizenship survey. Paper presented to Sustainable Economic Growth for Regional Australia (SEGRA) 5th National Conference, 10 - 12 September 2001, Townsville.

Stroeken, K. (2001), Defying the gaze: exodelics for the bewitched in Sukumaland and beyond. *Dialectical Anthropology* 26: 285-309.

Swift, J. (1989), Why are rural people vulnerable to famine. *IDS Bulletin,* 20(2) 8-15.

Swift, J. & K. Hamilton (2001), Household food security and livelihood security. In: S. Devereux & S. Maxwell (Eds.) *Food security in Sub-Saharan Africa*. London: ITDG Publishing, pp. 67-92.

Tanner, M., D. De Savigny, C. Mayornbana, C. Hatz, E. Burrüer, S. Tayari & A. Degremont (1991). Morbidity and mortality at Kilombero 1982-88. In: R.G. Feachern & D.T. Jamison (Eds.) *Disease and Mortality in Sub-Saharan Africa*. Oxford: Oxford University Press, pp. 286-305.

Tanzania Commission for AIDS (TACAIDS), National Bureau of Statistics (NBS), and ORC Marco (2005), *Tanzania HIV/AIDS Indicator Survey 2003-04*. Calverton, Maryland, USA: TACAIDS, NBS and ORS Marco.

Tarimo, E., M. Ntabaye & D. Simba (2003), *Towards a National quality framework: Experiences and Lessons*. Dar es Salaam: Ministry of Health.

Tibaijuka, A. (1997), AIDS and economic welfare in peasant agriculture: case studies from Kagabiro village Kagera Region, Tanzania. *World Development* 25: 963-75.

Tibandebage, P. & M. Mackintosh (2002), Institutional reform and regulatory relationships in a liberalising health care system: a Tanzanian case study. In: J. Heyer, R. Thorp & F. Stewart (Eds.) *Group Behaviour and Development*, Oxford: Oxford University Press, pp. 271-289.

Topouzis, D. (2000), *Measuring the impact of HIV/AIDS on the agricultural sector in Africa*. Geneva: UNAIDS.

Topouzis, D. & G. Hemrich (1996), The socio-economic impact of HIV/AIDS on rural families in Uganda. United Nations Development Programme *(UNDP) Discussion Paper No. 6*, New York: UNDP.

Tronto, J. (1993), *Moral Boundaries: A Political Argument for an Ethic of Care*. New York, London: Routledge.

Tumushabe, J. (2005), HIV/AIDS and the changing vulnerability to Crisis in Tanzania: Implications for food security and poverty eradication. A paper presented in the International Conference on HIV/AIDS, Food and Nutrition Security, April 14-16, 2005 Durban, South Africa.

United Kingdom office of National statistics (UKONS) (2001), *Social capital: A review of literature*. London: UKONS.

UNAIDS (1999), *A review of household and community responses to the HIV/AIDS epidemic in the rural areas of sub-Saharan Africa*. Geneva: UNAIDS.

UNAIDS (1999), *Gender and HIV/AIDS: Taking stock of research and programmes*. Geneva: UNAIDS.

UNAIDS (2000), *AIDS- Palliative care*. Geneva: UNAIDS.

UNAIDS (2001), *HIV/AIDS, Food Security, and Rural Development*. Geneva: UNAIDS.

UNAIDS & WHO (2006), *AIDS Epidemic update*. Geneva: UNAIDS.

UNAIDS, UNICEF & WHO (2004), *United Republic of Tanzania, Epidemiological Fact sheet on HIV/AIDS and sexually transmitted infections*. Geneva: UNAIDS

The United Nations Population Fund (UNFPA) (2005), *Tanzania Country Profiles for Population and Reproductive Health, Policy Developments and Indicators*. New York: UNFPA.

United Nations (1995), *Beijing Declaration and Platform for Action*. New York: United Nations.

Uphoff, N. & C.M. Wijayaratna (2000), Demonstrated benefits from social capital: the productivity of farmers organizations in Gal Oya, Sri Lanka. *World Development* 28(11): 1875-1890.

United Republic of Tanzania (1978), *Population and Housing Census.* Dar es Salaam: National Bureau of Statistics (NBS).

United Republic of Tanzania (1997), *The Agricultural Policy of Tanzania.* Dar es Salaam: Ministry of Agriculture.

United Republic of Tanzania (2000), *Poverty Reduction Strategy Paper*, Dar es Salaam: URT.

United Republic of Tanzania (2001), *National HIV/AIDS Policy*, Dar es Salaam: URT.

United Republic of Tanzania (2002), *Tanzania Household Budget Survey,* Dar es Salaam: National Bureau of Statistics (NBS).

United Republic of Tanzania (2003a), *2002 Population and Housing census,* Dar es salaam: National Bureau of Statistics (NBS).

United Republic of Tanzania (2003b), *National multi-sectoral strategic framework on HIV/AIDS 2003-07,* Dar es Salaam: The Prime Minister's Office, URT.

United Republic of Tanzania (2005a), *National HIV/AIDS Surveillance Report No 19.* Dar es Salaam: Ministry of Health (MOH).

United Republic of Tanzania (2005b) Survaillance of HIV/AIDS and syphilis infections among antenatal clinic attendees 2003/04. Dar es Salaam: Ministry of Health (MOH).

Vogel, C. & K. O'Brien (2004), *Vulnerability and global environment change: Rhetoric and Reality.* AVISO: An information bulletin on Global Environmental Change and Human Security project Issue No. 13. Victoria BC, Canada: GECHS.

Von Benda-Beckmann, F. & K. Von Benda-Beckmann (1994), Coping with insecurity. In: F. Von Benda-Beckmann, K. Von Benda-Beckmann & H. Marks (Eds.) Coping with insecurity: An underall perspective on social security in the Third World. *Focaal* 22/23:7-31.

Wallerstein, I. & J. Smith (1991), Households as institution of the world economy. In: R. L. Blumberg (Ed.) *Gender, Family and the Economy, the triple overlap.* Newbury Park: SAGE Publications, pp. 225-242.

Weissmann, M. (2005), Informal networks as a conflict preventive mechanism. In: L. P. Niklas Swanström (Ed.) *Conflict Prevention and Conflict Management in Northeast Asia.* Uppsala & Washington: CACI and SRSP, pp. 103-120.

Wellman, B. & S. Wortley (1989), Brothers' keepers: situating kinship relations in broader networks of social support. *Sociological Perspectives* 32: 273-306.

Wiegers, E., J. Curry, A. Garbero & J. Hourihan (2006), Patterns of vulnerability of AIDS impacts in Zambian Households. *Development and Change* 37(3): 1073-1092.

Wilkinson, R.G. (1996), *Unhealthy Societies: The Affliction of Inequality.* London: Routledge and Kagen Paul.

Wilkinson, R.G. (2002), Commentary: liberty, fraternity, equality. *International Journal of Epidemiology* 31: 538-543.

Winchester, P. (1992), *Power, Choice and Vulnerability: A Case Study in Disaster Mismanagement in South India.* London: James and James.

Wisner, B., P. Blaikie, T. Cannon & I. Davis (2004), *At Risk: Natural Hazards, People's Vulnerability and Disaster.* London: Routledge (2nd Edition).

Woolcock, M. (2000), Friends in high place? An overview of social capital. *Development Research Insights issue 34*. Brighton: Institute of Development Studies.

Woolcock, M. & D. Narayan (2000), Social capital: implication for development theory, research and policy. *World Bank Observer* 15: 225-249.

World Bank (1986), *Poverty and hunger: issues and option for food security in developing countries.* Washington DC: World Bank.

World Bank (1996), Social Capital. A report from a Working Group to the Task Force on Social Policy. Washington DC: World Bank.

World Bank (1997), *Confronting AIDS.* Washington DC and Oxford: World Bank and Oxford University.

World Bank (2000a), Intensifying action against HIV/AIDS in Africa: Responding to a development Crisis. Washington DC: World Bank.

World Bank (2000b), *World Development report 2000/2001: Attacking poverty*. New York. Oxford University Press for World Bank.

World Bank (2003), *World Development Indicators.* Washington DC: World Bank. World Bank poverty net website (Accessed on 16/12/2005: 2017).

Yin, R.K. (2003), *Case Study Research*. London, New Delhi: Sage Publication. (3rd edition).

Zak, P. & S. Knack (2001), Trust and Growth. *Economic Journal* 470(3): 295-321.

Appendix 1. Factors influencing household food security (N=180)

Explanatory variables	B-coefficient	Standard error
Age (years)	-0.0027325	0.01121
Household headship (1=male)	1.161896**	0.5845757
Education level (1=educated)	-0.1364458	0.3874667
Effective dependency ratio	-0.2377367	0.2023104
Marital status (1=married)	0.8874843*	0.4994547
HIV/AIDS status (1=affected)	0.0021078	0.4170249
Death/s in the household (1=yes)	-0.1603676	0.3456402
Estimated household annual income (Tshs)	8.08e-07***	3.02e-07
Land ownership (1=yes)	0.3006023	0.3167439
Sale of labour (1=yes)	1.660242***	0.3377689
Group membership (1=yes)	0.2525186	0.3089488
Support during illness (1=yes)	0.346285	0.5708413
Support during food shortage (1=yes)	-0.0024572	0.4068696

LR Chi^2 (13) = 54.13
Prob > Chi^2 = 0.000
Pseudo R^2 = 0.1402
Log likelihood = -165.9579

*p<0.10, **p<0.05 and ***p<0.01.
Source: Household Survey, 2005.

Summary

The role of social capital in development is receiving increasing attention. Indeed, social capital seems to have evolved into panacea for all problems affecting poor communities. The HIV/AIDS pandemic represents a serious threat to rural livelihood in Tanzania. The question is how social capital produced in social networks is used, generated and maintained in a context of HIV/AIDS. This study investigated HIV/AIDS impacts on social capital and their implications for rural livelihoods. The study moved beyond the household, by looking at the significance of social networks for the coping capacity of individuals and households. It emphasizes the ability of individuals and households to mobilize resources through social networks such as kinship networks, friends and neighbours, and community groups. A gender perspective was integrated into the research questions and study design. The study was conducted in Mkamba village, in Morogoro region in Tanzania. It used qualitative methods, such as key informants interviews, focus group discussions and in-depth case study interviews, as well as a household survey and group inventory.

Socio-economic information gathered from the area indicates a high level of livelihood insecurity. Although the sugarcane plantations and factories provide employment, the privatization of the sugar company has made many households vulnerable to poverty. Some who were employed in the factories lost their jobs, while those who still work in the factories do not earn sufficient income for a living. The sugar company reclaimed its legally owned land that was previously used by village inhabitants, thus forcing farming households to hire distant plots for the cultivation of food crops. Although households in the area are also engaged in other income-generating activities, these are constrained by lack of start-up capital and low local purchasing power. In-migration has increased ethnic diversity, which has contributed to a decline of trust among community members. Witchcraft beliefs and anti-witchcraft initiatives are widely common and part of social life in the study area, but also have a deteriorating effect on community trust.

This study was focused on the effects of HIV/AIDS on households and the community. The most direct impact of HIV/AIDS on households is the loss of human capital. HIV/AIDS-related morbidity and mortality affect households by reducing household time and labour and changing the responsibilities and time allocation of the household members. For HIV/AIDS-affected households it is difficult to pursue on-farm and off-farm activities since most of their resources are spent on immediate care requirements. As a result, they are unable to generate sufficient income. The HIV/AIDS-induced changes in the resource base of households jeopardize their food security. Although many households in the village face food insecurity in certain periods of the year, poor and HIV/AIDS-affected households were found to be chronically food insecure.

The HIV/AIDS epidemic affects different households in different ways and produces a variety of coping strategies. Faced with HIV/AIDS impacts and other stresses, households continuously pursue coping responses to counteract their detrimental effects. The HIV/AIDS epidemic has impoverished directly affected households. Once households lose their assets, their chances to recover and rebuild their livelihoods become slim. The household assets base was found to be an important determinant of the ability to cope with HIV/AIDS impacts. Strong links between HIV/AIDS and poverty is demonstrated, with HIV/AIDS exacerbating existing problems such as household food insecurity, while at the same time poverty increases vulnerability to HIV/AIDS impacts. Gender and age were found to be important attributes shaping HIV/AIDS impacts. Women are disproportionately affected. Female-headed households were found to have higher dependency ratios than male-headed ones. HIV/AIDS is placing a great burden on women who, in a situation of declining resources, care for the sick and other surviving members. Prime-age adult mortality undermines the livelihood sustainability of the ones left behind, especially elderly people and orphans.

It is generally expected that households that face difficulties try to secure support from others, like relatives, friends and neighbours. Extended families and kinship networks are regarded as the main source of social, economic and practical support for individuals. In the wake of HIV/AIDS and other socio-economic difficulties, kinship support was found to be hardly available. The context in which families provide support to their members has changed. Migration and the splitting-up of families have led to weakened family ties and declining transfers. Additionally, economic constraints limit the support one can get from relatives. In the study area kinship networks proved to be of little significance as providers of social support.

In a situation of geographical dispersal of extended family members, relations with friends and neighbours become an important source of social support. Beyond the immediate and extended family, households in crisis turn to friends and neighbours for assistance. However, the findings from this study show that support from friends and neighbours tends to be short-term and unreliable, usually limited to advice and emotional support. As a consequence of widespread poverty in the study area families are often too burdened with their own problems to be of much help to others. Witchcraft suspicion and accusations, while indicating deteriorating interpersonal trust, also create barriers to access support that might otherwise be provided by friends and neighbours. It was found that support to those with problems is hindered by fear of witchcraft suspicion and accusation. Stigma attached to HIV/AIDS limits the support one can get from neighbours and friends. Likewise, the secrecy surrounding HIV/AIDS limits the assistance from the community to those affected. It was found that social networks mobilized through interpersonal ties are not able to provide sufficient support to buffer the crises faced by most of the HIV/AIDS-affected households and other vulnerable households. HIV/AIDS affects households such that investing in social relationships becomes difficult, thereby excluding them from informal support mechanisms.

Several groups formed in the area help people manage different crises. It was found that the villagers participate in groups such as saving-and-credit groups, production groups, ethnic associations, and burial and festival groups, mostly for economic reasons but also for a sense of belonging and emotional or spiritual support. Most of the groups in the area were found to have financial constraints and assistance given to group members is too little to meet the demands of needy households. The local groups also lack access to information and resources from other social groups, which indicates a lack of bridging social capital. Despite the potential benefits of membership groups, the required contributions prevent some individuals from becoming members. Poor and HIV/AIDS-affected households are generally left out when it comes to participation in groups. It was found that social capital generated in formal groups benefit members only, rather than improving the welfare of the community as a whole. Community groups that strengthen social capital for some individuals lead to the exclusion of others.

There are clear differences in the type of groups to which men and women belong. Men dominate groups that produce substantial resources but also require significant initial financial contributions. Examples are the sugarcane out-grower production group and formally registered saving-and-credit groups. Generally, women groups have less status and influence than men groups. Although women groups in the study area service the poor, the very poor are left out because they cannot meet group membership qualifications. Most of the activities of these groups are aimed at providing resources for household well-being. Women's groups work for the improvement of women's living conditions but do not address the prevailing gender inequality.

In the study area, there has been hardly any community-level mobilization in response to the devastating effects of the HIV/AIDS epidemic. Funerals only are the communal events that display cooperation among community members. Although the socio-economic situation in the area has already weakened support relations, HIV/AIDS seems to have made matters worse. HIV/AIDS impacts exhaust the capacities and potential of a community. HIV/AIDS morbidity and mortality take away people who otherwise might have been involved in community activities. HIV/AIDS and other socio-economic problems put strains on households and communities to the extent that recourse to social capital becomes difficult. As individuals and households struggle to make ends meet, they have little time left for group and community activities and concerns.

The study found that inability to maintain social relations at the interpersonal level results in unintended collective effects at community level, such as lack of cooperation and trust among community members. Distrust at the interpersonal level is extended to the community level, preventing people to work together to solve their problems. In the study area, there was a general feeling that community solidarity and trust had declined during the past decades. Deteriorating trust is attributed to widespread poverty, ethnic diversity, and witchcraft suspicions and accusations. HIV/AIDS prevention, care and mitigation of its impacts proved to be difficult in a situation where there are multiple socio-economic problems as well as lack of community trust and solidarity. Therefore, the study underscores the importance of contextualizing the role of interpersonal and community-level social capital when studying HIV/AIDS impacts on livelihoods.

About the author

Carolyne Ignatius Nombo was born on 18th February 1969 in Musoma, Tanzania. She obtained a BSc. degree in Home Economics and Human Nutrition in 1993 and a MSc. degree in Agricultural Extension and Education in 1995 from Sokoine University of Agriculture, Morogoro, Tanzania.

She started her professional career in October 1995 as the first coordinator of an NGO known as *Mtandao wa Vikundi vya Wakulima Tanzania* - MVIWATA (Tanzania Farmers Groups Network). From 1998 she worked as country representative of INTERMON OXFAM an international NGO dealing with livelihood and development programs. She represented INTERMON OXFAM in various fora and facilitated local partners in the conception, implementation, monitoring and evaluation of various livelihood projects. She then became technical advisor for a community-based food security program in the regions of Morogoro and Dodoma. In this capacity, she provided overall support to program management issues by offering inputs to key managerial processes such as strategic planning, review and evaluation.

In 2003 she obtained a sandwich scholarship through the AWLAE Project to pursue her PhD with the Sociology of Consumers and Households Group at Wageningen University and Research Centre. Her research areas of interest include rural livelihoods, community-based initiatives and gender issues.

She is married and mother of two sons.